Creepy Crawly
CUISINE

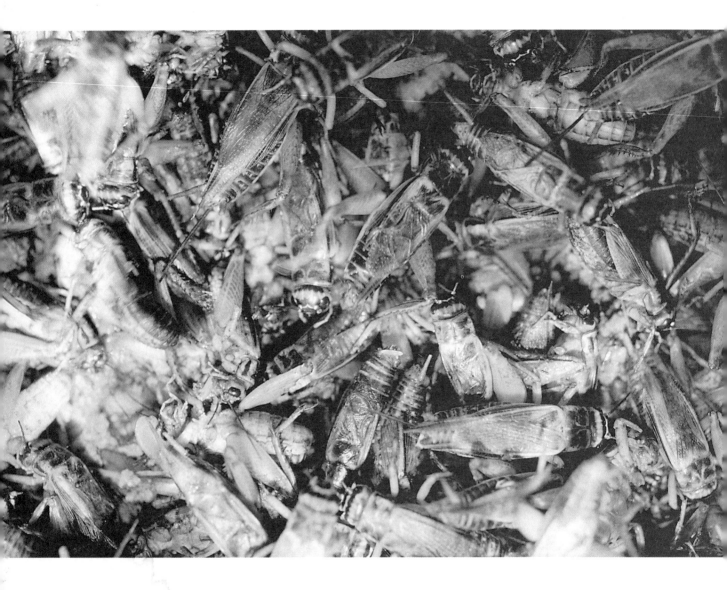

Creepy Crawly
CUISINE

The Gourmet Guide to Edible Insects

Julieta Ramos-Elorduy, Ph.D.

Translated from the Spanish by Nancy Esteban

Park Street Press
Rochester, Vermont

To whom is manifested inside the invisible at every moment

Park Street Press
One Park Street
Rochester, Vermont 05767
www.gotoit.com

Library of Congress Cataloging-in-Publication Data
Ramos-Elorduy, Julieta.
    Creepy crawly cuisine : the gourmet guide to edible insects / Julieta Ramos-Elorduy ; photographs by Peter Menzel.
        p.   cm.
    Includes bibliographical references.
    ISBN 0-89281-747-X   (pbk. : alk. paper)
    1. Cookery (Insects). 2. Edible insects. I. Menzel, Peter, 1948– . II. Title.
TX746.R36   1998   97-48506
641.6'96—dc21   CIP

Printed and bound in Canada

10 9 8 7 6 5 4 3 2 1

Text design by Virginia L. Scott
This book was typeset in Goudy and Lucida Sans

Special thanks to Chris Kilham for his inspired title.

Park Street Press is a division of Inner Traditions International

Distributed to the book trade in Canada by Publishers Group West (PGW), Toronto, Ontario
Distributed to the book trade in the United Kingdom by Deep Books, London
Distributed to the book trade in Australia by Millennium Books, Newtown, N.S.W.
Distributed to the book trade in New Zealand by Tandem Press, Auckland
Distributed to the book trade in South Africa by Alternative Books, Ferndale

Contents

Soups

Main Courses

Sauces

Desserts

Foreword

Professor Julieta Ramos-Elorduy has probably contributed more to our knowledge of edible insects than has any other person, past or present. For more than twenty years, she and able colleagues at the National Autonomous University in Mexico have studied the use of insects as food in the Mexican countryside. Such use of insects dates to the precolumbian times, and the Mexican researchers have documented use of more than two hundred species. That total is far greater than documented in any other country, though the use of insect foods is not unique to Mexico. In most countries in Africa, southern and eastern Asia, and northern sections of South America, dozens of insect species are among the traditional foods.

Historically (and prehistorically for that matter) insects have played an important role in global nutrition. Early travelers to Africa noted that populations that had access to termites and locusts were in noticeably better condition than those that had no access. In fact, the appearance of a locust swarm was viewed with joy by those who did not have crops at risk. In some ways, things haven't changed much. Newspapers in Zimbabwe reported that when grasshoppers unexpectedly invaded the suburbs of the capital city of Harare, "Housewives abandoned their domestic chores to fetch buckets, bottles and tins to fill them with the delicious insects."

Insects have not been used merely to ward off starvation. They have held an esteemed place in the cuisines of many countries. A modern cookbook on Cameroon cuisine describes the recipe for "coconut larvae" as "a favorite dish offered only to good friends." Coconuts at the half-hard stage are emptied of their milk, refilled with the larvae and condiments, then cooked (capped end up) in water.

Dr. Ramos-Elorduy and her colleagues have conducted extensive studies in the nutrient content of edible insects. Live insects contain about the same amount of protein as other animals, but in the dried form frequently found in village markets they are very high in protein—and the protein is of high quality, especially when used in combination with other foods. Insects vary in their fat content, some being high in fat (fortunate for those who need more calories), others being low in fat (fortunate for those who are watching their calories). And to the benefit of everyone, insect fatty acids are highly unsaturated, being comparable to those of fish and poultry. Insects are a good source of many of the important vitamins and minerals, including thiamin (vitamin B_1), riboflavin (B_2), iron, and zinc. Dr. Ramos-Elorduy has researched the nutrients furnished by insects within the context of Mexico's staple foods and nutritional needs. She has proclaimed the high biological efficiency of some insects in protein production (their high food conversion efficiency and high reproductive capacity) and the fact that some insects utilize food substrates that are otherwise poorly utilized in food production. These attributes of insects when used as food have important global environmental ramifications.

The "age of edible insects" may just be dawning. While they have long been traditional foods in many cultures, a new wave of interest is sweeping through the Western world, evidenced by the favorable attention being given to edible insects by the Western media. Also, as the former editor of *The Food Insects Newsletter*, I regularly received letters from U.S. readers asking to know where they could find recipes, where they could find edible wild insects, or where they could purchase insect delicacies imported from other countries.

Edible insects are also making inroads into the Western academic community, being included in introductory biology courses, ranging from those in elementary schools to others at the university level. A new entomology textbook published in London by Australian authors devotes an entire section to edible insects. In 1992 the New York Entomological Society celebrated its 100th anniversary by holding a "bug banquet" at the staid Explorers Club in New York City. The speaker of the evening used the title, "Insects are Food: Where Has the Western World Been?" So, the so-called West may be now awakening to what it has been missing and soon be joining Mexico and the rest of the world in using and enjoying this vast and varied food resource.

Gene R. DeFoliart
Professor Emeritus
University of Wisconsin—Madison
December 1997

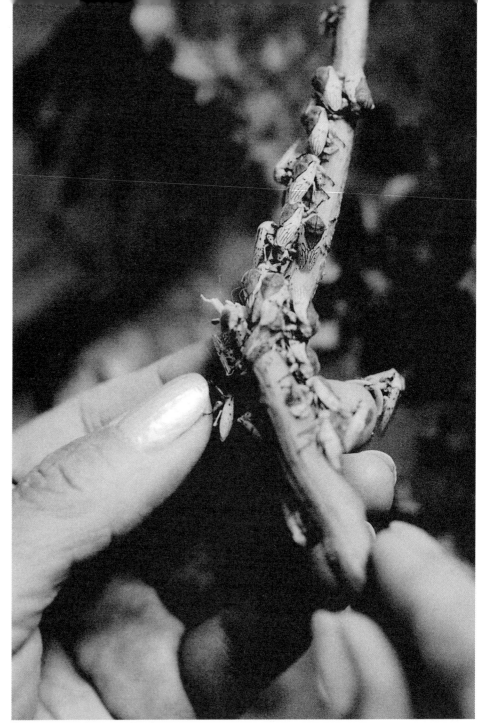

CHAPTER 1

Introduction

Preparing treehoppers for the pot

INSECTS ANYONE?

For many people the idea of actually eating insects may seem incredible, perhaps even shocking. And while for these people insects may seem a strange choice of nourishment, for millions of human beings throughout the world insects constitute a daily food vital to their existence. It is surprising that an animal group as abundant and nutritious as insects remains such an underutilized resource, not only by those living in urban areas, but by some of those in rural communities as well. The negative (and mostly false) perception of insects as being disease-ridden and dirty has prevented a good number of cultures from taking advantage of a delicious, protein-packed food source. Few people know that insects are actually closely related to lobsters and shrimp—they belong to the same phylum—and that in reality they are as tasty and appealing as their well known, but more expensive, crustacean cousins.

To date 1,417 species of edible insects have been recorded in the world and the number of ethnic groups partaking in the consumption of insects (known as *entomophagy*) stands close to 3,000. Those included in this group range from inhabitants of the deserts of Africa to the countryside of Asia to the urban centers of the United States. The edible species are comprised of fifteen orders of insects—Anoplura (lice), Orthoptera (grasshoppers, crickets, and cockroaches), Hemiptera (true bugs), Homoptera (cicadas and treehoppers), Hymenoptera (bees, ants, and wasps), Diptera (flies and mosquitoes), Coleoptera (beetles), Lepidoptera (butterflies and moths), Megaloptera (alderflies and dobsonflies), Odonata (dragonflies and damselflies), Ephemeroptera (mayflies), Trichoptera (caddisflies), Plecoptera (Stoneflies), Neuroptera (lacewings and antlions) and Isoptera (termites)—and are distributed in 112 families, 628 genera, 45 subgenera and 67 subspecies. The majority of edible insects are most frequently eaten in their larval and pupal stages.

JUST WHAT ARE INSECTS?

It might surprise most people to know that insects are the predominant animal group on earth, constituting four-fifths of the animal kingdom. They have inhabited the earth for more than 300 million years—compared to man's brief existence of only one million years—and have evolved and adapted to an amazing variety of habitats, demonstrating highly developed social organizations. Because of their miraculous ability to adapt, insects have conquered practically all existing habitats worldwide, even such unlikely environments as pools of petroleum and salt mines. They can be found in trees and shrubs, on the ground, in roots, in the sand, and in an array of aquatic environments. What other animal group shows such remarkable versatility?

Generally speaking, we think of insects as small pesky animals that move, jump, leap, eat, fly, and bite—but from a more scientific standpoint, just what *is* an insect?

Insects are animals belonging to the phylum Arthropoda, which means they have limbs or articulated appendages. This phylum includes spiders, mites, members of the cheliceral class and, as mentioned before, shrimp, lobsters, and crabs.

TABLE 1

Species of edible insects recorded worldwide.

Lice	3
Mayflies	7
Dragonflies	20
Grasshoppers, cockroaches, & crickets	239
Termites	39
True bugs	92
Cicadas and little cicadas	73
Scorpionflies	4
Butterflies and Moths	235
Stick carrier	5
Flies and mosquitoes	3
Beetles	344
Ants, bees, and wasps	313
Total	**1,417**

While there are exceptions to the rules, insects are usually small in size, more or less elongated, almost always cylindrical, and of bilateral symmetry. Their bodies are segmented into three regions: the head, which carries the buccal parts (mouth), eyes, ocelli, and antenna; the thorax, which incorporates the legs (three pairs) and the wings (two pairs, when present); and the abdomen, which carries modified appendages that make up the genitalia. As a general rule, most of the appendages are segmented.

In contrast to man, whose bones are located internally, an insect's support structure—known as the exoskeleton—is found outside its body. Insects' breathing is conducted through branching tubes called tracheae that take oxygen directly to the cells without the use of lungs. Insects possess compound eyes, giving them a mosaic vision, and some species are mimetic, enabling them to imitate not only the form but the color of the substratum in which they live. Another distinguishing characteristic of insects is that they are cold-blooded; their body temperatures vary from below freezing to more than 86° Fahrenheit.

Those insects most commonly consumed by human beings fall into the following categories: beetles (Coleoptera); grasshoppers and crickets (Orthoptera); butterflies and moths (Lepidoptera); bees, wasps and ants (Hymenoptera); true bugs (Hemiptera); and dragonflies (Odonata). The appearance of these insects varies greatly and their tastes can range from nutty to lemony to shrimplike. As one might expect, geography plays a significant role in the amount and the type of insects consumed.

A Brief History

While dining on insects may seem a relatively new idea—a part of the "alternative" movement gaining popularity throughout the world—the fact is that using insects as a food source is an idea that has been around for hundreds of thousands of years. It is only recently that some industrialized nations have begun to view entomophagy as a viable option, but cave drawings and other records from ancient civilizations reveal that insects were a part of the cuisine of our ancestors. From the beginning of humankind's existence, we have used insects and their by-products, not only for sustenance but in our medicinal treatments and religious rituals as well.

In Mexico such indigenous tribes as the Mayans referred to locusts of the *Schistocerca* genus as "the divine flowers of God"; the pupal stage of some wood worm beetles are known by the Lacandones as "little virgins." The Huicholes believed various species of wasps acted as bearers of the souls of the dead to the heavens, and among the Teotihuacans, the butterfly of the *Papilio daunus* species called *Xochiquetzal* was considered the soul itself!

For generations insects have been used in folk medicine as treatments for various types of illness and diseases. Today insects continue to be used live, cooked, ground, in infusions, and in salves. In many Eastern European countries insects are a common tool in modern medicine. In fact, in countries that until recently existed behind the Iron Curtain entire hospitals are dedicated to using different bee products through inhalation, ionization, physiotherapy, and electrophoresis. Recently, leafcutting ants have been used in the operating room to close wounds. The ants, whose jaws act as surgical clamps, not only join the wound but also induce scarring. Infection is even prevented by the bactericidal substances produced by the mandibular glands of ants of the *Atta* genus.

Extracts from insects have been used to treat urogenital and liver disease. The chitin derived from the exoskeleton of insects is used as a treatment for lowering cholesterol and repairing tissue, as an anticoagulant, and as an agent that accelerates scarring and works against pathogens in the blood or on the skin. It is also used as a carrier of medicinal substances. It is even used to fabricate contact lenses!

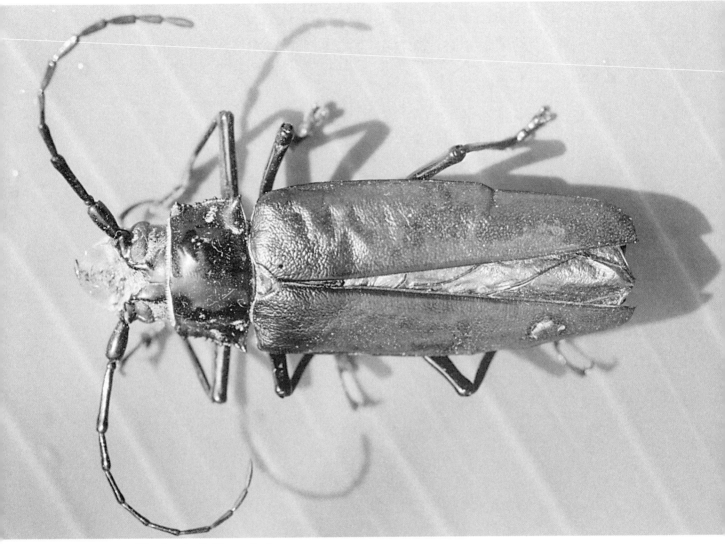

The beetle *Callipogon barbatum*

A Bad Rap

Considering the multitude of ways people benefit from insects, it is curious that insects continue to suffer from such an unfavorable reputation. The irony is that while many of us perceive insects as harmful pests—dangerous, ugly, and disease ridden—in reality, without the service of pollination which they provide humankind might cease to exist. The promotion of negative stereotypes of insects can be largely traced to failure by Europeans to appreciate or understand the customs of the lands they colonized and their misperception that the way of life of most indigenous populations they encountered was barbaric. Many people's dislike for insects stems from a similar classist attitude that associates insects with indigenous people who lack the means to buy or grow alternate sources of food. Again this prejudice stems largely from Western cultures. In contrast, cultures of many Eastern nations such as Japan and China consider various species of insects to be great delicacies.

Historically speaking, some species of insects have been the cause of serious economic loss—especially of food supply, which has promoted both the idea of insects as a blight and the popularity of the often repeated biblical reference "a plague of locusts." But in modern times there is no greater culprit than humankind for perpetuating the bad name of insects. Through our agricultural practices we have modified the world environment and ecosystem, providing a surplus food supply to the insect world, thereby inducing their proliferation. In hope of protecting our food supplies, insecticides were used—first natural substances and later synthetic ones—and as a result resistant strains of insects have developed while we continue to poison ourselves and our environment with stronger and more deadly toxins.

THE ROAD AHEAD

It may be a considerable amount of time before noninsect-eating cultures are able to put aside their prejudices, roll up their sleeves, and dig into the culinary delights of cooking with insects. But signs are beginning to emerge that times are changing. Not only do cultures traditionally known for eating insects continue to do so, but momentum is growing throughout the rest of the world's population to join them. For this we can thank publications such as *The Food Insects Newsletter,* and businesses such as Hot Lix, a novelty candy company in California that sells such products as Cricket Lick-It—Creme-de-Menthe-flavored suckers with a cricket at the center—and AMBER InsectNside—a toffee flavored, brittle-style candy with insects trapped inside to give it the look of genuine fossilized amber. So whether you roast them, marinate them, butter-fry them, or dip them in chocolate, insects may not remain a foreign food for long!

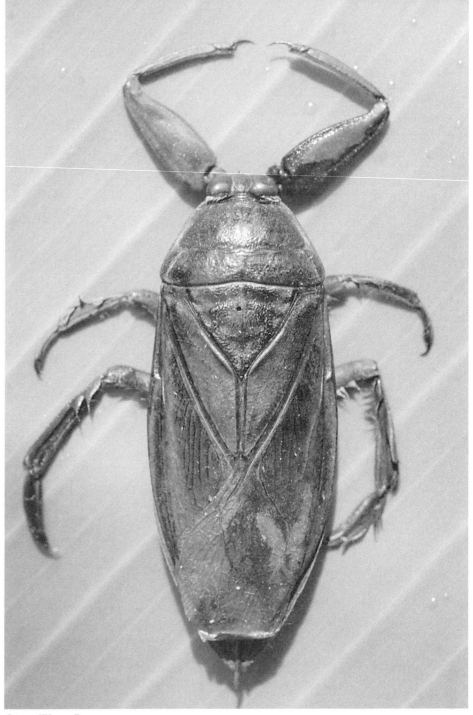

CHAPTER TWO

Entomophagy Around the World

Giant Water Bug

The Worldwide Web

Keeping in mind that there are an estimated 300 to 400 million species of insects in the world, it seems probable that there may be thousands, perhaps millions, more edible insects than the 1,417 species recorded to date. Because of their great diversity and range of locale, only a small portion of the entire insect family has been studied and determined fit for consumption. And yet, throughout the thousands of years that human beings have eaten insects, remarkably few cases of illness have been associated with such a diet. People from all corners of the world practice entomophagy, but the frequency and culinary creativity with which insects are used varies greatly in species from one country to the next, though their preparation and use are often similar.

Which insects are used as food depends on a variety of factors: season, location, and especially the amount of time and energy required to harvest certain species. Some insects might be quite delicious, but the task of collecting them is not always a simple matter and in some cases extremely difficult.

The most commonly consumed insects are those species that live in large, densely grouped populations which are easily and quickly collected and found in convenient locations. Insects considered to be "social"—such as bees, wasps, ants, and termites—or those that exhibit some type of herd instinct or develop in groups—like butterflies and tree worms, respectively—are the insects most often eaten.

FLAVOR AND APPEARANCE

As might be expected, taste is the principal criterion determining which insects are considered most edible. Insects vary greatly in flavor. Some, such as wasps, taste similar to pine nuts, while stink bugs have a pleasant applelike flavor (see chart on opposite page). Depending on your preference (as well as your resources), insects can be eaten live, roasted, or mixed into dishes such as rice, soup, salads, and pasta. They can be used as a topping for pizza or even as a garnish for mixed drinks! Different cultures prepare similar insects in a variety of ways to increase their palatability.

In gauging the palatability of insects, other important *organoleptic* criteria—those pertaining to the senses—are appearance, smell, and texture.

But, as with so many other foods, an insect's pleasing color is not always indicative of a pleasant taste. Generally, the color of an insect serves to identify the species or to differentiate between it and another in the same family: the red wasp, the black bee, the yellow tail, the green worm, the black cricket. In fact the larvae and pupae of most insects either are white or lack any color at all. Because the majority of edible insects are ingested in their immature stage, they are more often identified by form than by color. For example, the butterfly *Sinopsia mexicanaria*, which is eaten in the Valle de Mexico, is called "little fish" not for its silver coloring, but because its larvae live in groupings like schools of fish and because it has a cocoon that resembles a fishing net.

During the cooking process insects such as grasshoppers undergo the same phenomenon that occurs with most crustaceans—their color changes from a

Flavors

Ants—sweet, almost nutty

Black witch moth larvae—herring

Central agave worms—kidney bean

Corn earworms—corn on the cob

Crickets and grasshoppers—mild, taking on surrounding flavors

Dragonfly larvae and other aquatic insect larvae—fish

Leaf-footed bugs—very sweet pumpkin

Nopal worms—fried potato

Red agave worms—spicy

Stinkbugs—apple

Termites—nutty

Tree worms—pork rinds

Treehoppers—from avocado to fried zuchini

Wasps—pine nuts

Water boatmen (adults)—fish (when fresh), shrimp (when dried)

Water boatmen and backswimmer eggs—caviar

White agave worms—cracklings

Yellow mealworm beetle larvae—whole wheat bread

natural gray, blue, or brown to a more appetizing red. If insects possessing large quantities of fat, like tree worms, are not prepared immediately after they are harvested, their fat will oxidize upon contact with air, turning them black. While this state does not affect their taste, it certainly decreases their visual appeal.

Because of their exoskeleton most insects give off very little odor and, therefore, smell has little influence on palatability. Conversely, this same shell greatly influences texture. Insects are crunchy and the act of chewing, coupled with the resulting salivation, carries with it great oral satisfaction, similar to the pleasure of eating pretzels or crackers. The exoskeleton is chewable and is actually an excellent source of fiber.

A last criterion often used for judging food is its nutritional value, and herein lies possibly the most persuasive argument for increasing the amount of crickets and ants in your diet. Insects are an extremely rich source of protein and minerals, and some have a high fat content, fat that can be transformed into energy. This makes them a particularly attractive food source for developing nations where protein is not as readily available as it is in more industrialized countries such as the United States and Canada. Nutrition, specifically the role insects can play in a healthy diet, will be discussed in greater detail in a later chapter.

WHY EAT INSECTS?

In both rural and urban areas of many developing nations, hunger and malnutrition continue to be significant problems. The insufficient intake of food-energy by many people is due, in part, to the lack of available sources of fats. Edible insects, especially those found in tree trunks, like tree worms, contain large amounts of fats that supply valuable calories that, in turn, can be converted into energy. This may not be considered beneficial in a society obsessed with low-fat foods, such as the United States, but in less affluent societies such sources of nutrients may provide the best means for avoiding malnutrition or even starvation.

For various tribes in the Amazon, tree worms are a primary source of dietary fat and essential calories. These worms are removed from tree trunks, cut lengthwise, then hung over receptacles on the fire; the dripping fat is collected and used to fry their meals. The worms are crisped and eaten in much the same way we eat pork rinds.

Ironically, while in many Western nations entomophagy remains the practice of the indigenous people, in others (in both the East and West) it has taken on the trappings of exclusivity, the practice of the upper class who view the eating of certain insects as a great delicacy. Today insects are exported to major cities around the world, including Tokyo, Paris, San Francisco, and New York, and sold at incredible prices in gourmet food shops. Different species are sold in assorted varieties, chocolate-covered ants, fried or chocolate-covered caterpillars, bees in syrup, and fried grasshoppers being only a few examples.

In Mexico City, the market price of some edible insects is commonly much higher than that of many meats! A pound of ants costs ten times more than a pound of meat, and the white agave worm fourteen times more. Grasshoppers, the red agave worm, and water boatmen eggs all cost twice the price of beef. As a consequence, the cost of a dish of insects prepared in a restaurant is often quite exorbitant. It may surprise some people to know that insect-eating traditions exist in Europe, too. In Puy de Dôme, France, and Sardinia, certain cheeses in which the fly larvae *Piophila casei* develop are considered a great delicacy, as are meats which have been infested by certain other types of flies.

In the majority of entomophagous countries insects are also preserved in vacuum-sealed jars and exported to nations with large immigrant or expatriate populations, as is the case with edible insects shipped from Turkey to Antwerp and sold to Turks who have gone there in search of employment.

TABLE 2

Number of edible insects per continent and number of consumer countries

Continent	No. of Species Recorded	%	Entomophagous Countries	%
Africa	527	36.04	36	31.86
America	573	39.14	23	20.00
Asia	249	17.03	29	25.60
Australia	86	5.88	14	12.39
Europe	27	1.86	11	9.73
Total	1,462*	100.00	113	100.00

* Some species occur on more than one continent, hence, this number is higher than 1,417.

FOREIGN FOOD

Just what are some of the places you might visit on a bug-eating excursion and what types of insects might you expect to eat? Believe it or not there are 113 entomophagous nations in the world, so it is likely that in your next visit abroad you'll have the chance, especially if you're looking, to come across a diverse selection of edible arthropods.

On the streets of Bangkok you can buy—among other things—a bag of fried grasshoppers, and on the coast of Macao fried cockroaches are sold in much the same way. Occasionally, grasshoppers and crickets there are even eaten raw.

During locust plagues in northern regions of Africa, locusts are caught in large steel drums which are then sealed for later use. In other parts of Africa, insects are dried on grills and later mixed with yucca flour and water, placed in plantain leaves or the leaves of another aromatic plant, and cooked in hot ashes. The forests of Central Africa produce a tremendous diversity of moth species that are eaten as caterpillars or are shipped to European capitals, where they are sold to immigrants from such countries as Congo and the Central African Republic.

In Japan the larvae of many aquatic insects are sold in supermarkets, skewered through the head, ten per skewer, six skewers per package. Insects such as the larvae of the wasp *Vespula lewisi*, the pupae of the silkworm known as *kaiko*, and the rice grasshopper *hashi* are canned in individual portions. Gift baskets of grasshoppers and crickets can be purchased in Japan much the way a basket of fruit is in the United States.

In Latin America sun-dried insects—grasshoppers, stink bugs, crickets, leaf-footed bugs, and beetles—are placed in sacks from which smaller portions are taken out as necessary and added to tacos and chili sauce, put in tortillas, or mixed in eggs, soups, or with shrimp and clams in rice. The larvae of beetles of the genus *Golopha*, a parasite of potato and chili crops, are much sought after in

Ecuador where they are collected with nets, sun-dried, then deposited in large tins. In Brazil, the tree worms and various stingless bees and wasps are known for their exquisite almondy taste.

In Columbia the culonas ants—especially the newly emerged queens—are enjoyed for their light nutty flavor. Like termites, these winged ants are collected with large sweeping brooms, placed immediately in boiling water, then taken out and dried on the grill. In the United States it is popular to dip the worker ants of this species in chocolate.

The Eskimos of Alaska eat the larvae of reindeer parasites (Oestridae), and in the western United States the larvae of the moth *Coloradia pandora* are collected and eaten. Native American tribes in California and Nevada set fire around the pine trees in which these larvae reside and then gather the larvae as they fall to the ground.

THE MOST POPULAR EDIBLE INSECTS

The introduction touched briefly upon the categories of the most commonly consumed insects, but now that we have a clearer understanding of entomophagy it may be interesting to learn a little more about these groups and where they are most often found.

Beetles (Coleoptera): There are twenty-four families of edible beetles recorded in the world and of these almost 50% are comprised of the long-horned beetle (Cerambycidae) and june, dung, and rhinoceros beetles (Scarabaeidae). Human communities living closest to forests—both tropical and temperate—make the most use of the beetle family as food, in that many beetles are wood borers readily found in living trees, fallen logs, and elsewhere on the floor of the forest. Sometimes several species coexist in the same tree trunk. They are highly efficient at transforming the indigestible (to humans) cellulose of the trees into digestible fat. One family of aquatic beetle, the Dytiscidae, is found in temperate as well as tropical waters and is widely consumed in Asia. The taste of most beetle larvae is similar to fried pork rinds. In the pupae state flavor is more concentrated, and in adults females are much tastier then males. Those coming from aquatic environments have a fishy flavor.

Butterflies and moths (Lepidoptera): Among those families of edible butterflies and moths (twenty-three in total), the nocturnal species are the most preferred, the most succulent and diversified of these belonging to the Saturniidae. This family makes up more than 50% of the moth species that man ingests, always in the larval (caterpillar) or pupal (cocoon) stages. The greatest numbers of lepidopterans are eaten in Africa where many species are dried, stored, and sold to international gastronomic markets. Caterpillars are high in both protein and iron, which makes consumption a major benefit in regions of Africa where children and pregnant women often suffer from deficiencies of both of these. The taste of butterflies and moths depends on the species and on the environment in which they are found, as well as on the manner of preparation. Roasted, fried, or boiled in salt water, some taste similar to chicken, others like codfish and herring. The most flavorful are those that bore into wood, which have the highest fat content.

The white agave worm is one of the most sought after of all edible insects. It lives in the leaves of the maguey agave plant, from which "honey water" and "pulque" drinks are made. The red agave worm is commonly found at the bottom of bottles of mescal as well, though this is not, of course, its natural environment. There is no cultivation of the white agave worm, as is the case with other species of edible insects. This is an issue that should receive attention because the price of one kilogram of them is an astounding $32 to $35. Such prices indicate a great market for this edible insect, which can reach lengths of four inches and widths

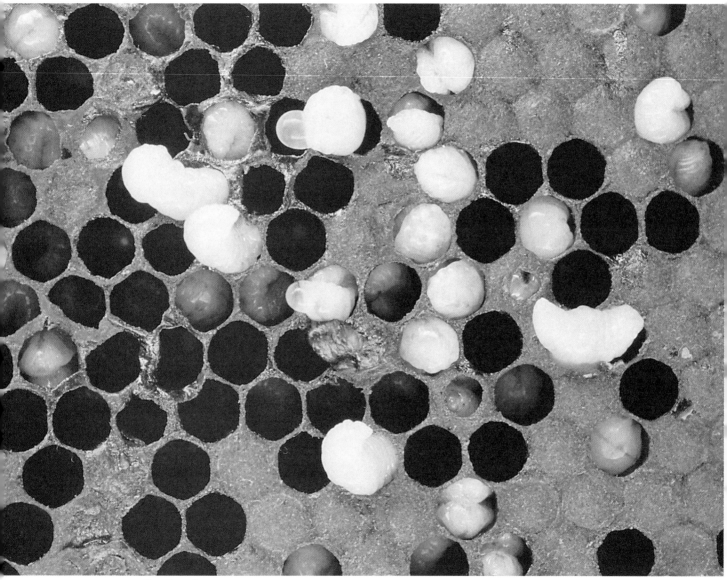

Bee brood

of two-thirds of an inch. Gourmet restaurants in Mexico City charge $15 for an entree of ten larvae, of which only half are authentic, the others being larvae of less desirable species such as nopal worm.

Bees, wasps, and ants (Hymenoptera): The biodiversity in bees, wasps, and ants is not as great as in that of some other insect groups. They are comprised of only eight significant families—three of bees, three of wasps, one ant, and the bumblebee. The immature stages of many species are used as food by indigenous people in Africa, Asia, Australia, South America, and Mexico. The stingless bees (Meliponidae) constitute 53% of the total edible Hymenoptera, with wasps coming in a distant second at 25%. Wasps are known for their pine-nutty flavor and the light, crystalline honey they produce. Many types of ants are popular food sources in South America. The brood of bees has a peanutty flavor or sometimes tastes like pine nuts or almonds. Ants are almost always nutty.

The yellow-tailed wasp inhabits tropical forests and is known for the elongated form of its honeycomb. In Mexico, the young of these wasps, as well as their honey, are highly regarded, and it is not unusual to see at least one nest of yellow-tailed wasps hanging in the home, scars on the hive indicating where cuts were made to extract the honey. These wasps are found throughout the American tropics, where they usually suspend their nests from palm trees.

Grasshoppers, crickets, and locusts. (Orthoptera): In this group, it is the grasshoppers (Acrididae) whose ten families make up 60% of the edible biomass. Grasshoppers are the most consumed type of insect due to their wide geographic distribution, diverse species, and the ease with which they can be caught and preserved. They are generally green, coffee-colored, or gray and turn an appealing red when boiled or fried. In Thailand, collecting grasshoppers and selling them has become an attractive alternative to reducing their population through often ineffective pesticide spraying. The flavor of grasshoppers and crickets is neutral and largely depends on how they are served, much as chicken does. Locusts, large insects responsible for what is known as the "plague of the locusts," are often found in "sleeves" whipping over large areas of vegetation, causing devastation. Famous for their frequent mention throughout the Bible, in some regions these insects are guarded and preserved. In the Koran, Muhammad denotes an obligation to eat these insects. Many different species of locust are eaten all over the world. Like grasshoppers, they do not have their own distinct flavor, but take on that of the sauce used.

Flies and Mosquitoes (Diptera): Edible flies and mosquitoes are represented by eleven families worldwide. The number of species making up these families is small, contrary to the true bugs (Hemiptera), which, in spite of a low number of families, have numerous species. Some orders, such as termites (Isoptera) and lice (Anoptura), are represented by only one family. Flies that develop on various kinds of cheese adopt the flavor of that cheese. Those from water environments can have a flavor like duck, and mosquitoes, when fresh, taste similarly to fish.

Water Boatmen and Backswimmers. These aquatic members of the order Hemiptera (true bugs) live in almost any kind of water—pure, stagnant, crystalline, alkaline—and species vary depending on habitat. They deposit their eggs on the stems of aquatic plants or on any object introduced into their environment, a quality that makes them an easy insect to cultivate and harvest. The eggs, known as Mexican caviar, are consumed after they have been dried and shaken off the plants they infest. In their fresh state they taste similarly to fish; when dried they taste more like shrimp.

Stink Bugs. These terrestrial members of Hemiptera are found in diverse ecosystems, but primarily in forests of pines and oaks under great layers of humus. This family is so famous in Mexico that a temple in Cerro del Huitzteco, in Taxco, is dedicated to it. On the first Monday following the Day of the Dead in November, there is a festival in this insect's honor, where a *señorita día del jumil* (Miss Stink Bug!) is elected. A scepter with a great stink bug sculpted in jade is presented to the young lady. These insects impart an exquisite apple taste when added to sauces and they are valued because they possess great amounts of iodine in an area where there is a serious lack of it. They also possess substances that have anesthetic and analgesic effects.

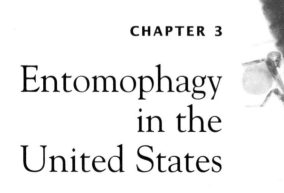

CHAPTER 3

Entomophagy in the United States

Dragonfly nymphs, *Aeshna multicolor*

Beetle Mania

When we think of foods associated with the United States, insects are not usually the first things that come to mind. Preservative-laden fast foods from such places as McDonalds, Burger King, or Taco Bell better fit the commercially-hyped stereotype of U.S. cuisine. But of course this diet of culinary convenience has not always been the standard. In fact, the United States (as well as many of its people) has a long record of entomophagy. To get a clearer picture of this we must consider the history of the first inhabitants of North America—people who came across the Bering Strait from Asia, people who would later diversify and are known today as Native Americans.

Overview

Native American cultures have a relationship with nature similar to that of many Asian countries—one of respect for and appreciation of nature's bounty. Traditionally, Native Americans have viewed the earth as a partner, not as an adversary, and for thousands of years before the arrival of Europeans on this continent, they both consumed and deified several insect species. There are numerous examples of native tribes whose diet included such insects as grasshoppers, ants, and caterpillars. The Pima Indians collected the caterpillars of the *Macrosita carolina* moth (known as the tobacco worm) and the *Coloradia pandora* to consume fried or to add in soups. The Assiniboine served up platefuls of pulverized ants and sun-dried locusts and grasshoppers, and the Shoshone ate crickets, grasshoppers, and ants.

With the discovery of the New World and its subsequent colonization, Europeans introduced to the Americas a very different view of the natural world—a view that saw nature as the enemy, a power capable of overwhelming and defeating them. With such an attitude it is not surprising that the colonists looked with suspicion on the native population's use of insects as food. Badly prepared to handle the difficulties of a new frontier, the colonists saw everything in the New World as a source of danger, especially something as inconceivable as eating insects! Threatened by the differences between Native Americans and themselves, most Europeans classified the natives as barbaric, a less civilized people. Consequently, insects came to be known pejoratively as "Indian food," the food of the savages.

This is not to say that insects were never consumed by European immigrants and their descendants. On the contrary, there are a number of recorded instances of entomophagy in the United States, especially in the western part of the country where, because of limited rainfall and less agricultural and economic development, hunger was more prevalent than in the East. In his book *Human Food Uses* Freeman cites a 1777 report describing captured French troops at West Point eating grasshoppers cooked on brochettes with great gusto. A report out of Utah in 1855 tells how, after locusts had devoured all the crops, the hungry inhabitants proceeded to eat the locusts! And, although such entomophagy was born of necessity rather than choice, there is no denying that insects did play a significant role in the diet of early European Americans.

Entomophagy was also practiced in the South, particularly among African slaves, a population that came from some of the most entomophagous locations in the world. It is easy to picture the slaves, horribly overworked and underfed, supplementing their inadequate protein intake by collecting grasshoppers in the field. With the liberation of the slaves at the end of the Civil War came a greater visibility of the use of insects as food in the emerging American culture.

AGRICULTURE AND INSECTS

Technology, especially in regard to agriculture, has been another significant deterrent to the practice of entomophagy in the United States. In tandem with the growth in agriculture and the U.S. population's dependence on it came a growth in the insect population, which now had a much larger food supply available to it. Insects such as locusts and boll weevils, at times responsible for destroying entire crops, affected not only the quantity but also the appearance of goods brought to market. Having grown accustomed to increasingly insect-free produce, Americans were no longer willing to purchase food infested with bugs. During this period, the perception of insects as an unhealthy food source continued to increase, while the population of North America's indigenous peoples—the primary communities practicing entomophagy—was restricted and reduced as the United States expanded westward, further limiting the practice of eating insects.

Accompanying the increase in domestic agricultural development was a declining reliance on wild animals as a primary food source. In place of wild game, Americans became increasingly dependent on domestic animals such as chickens, pigs, and cattle for their main source of food. Undoubtedly, this gave rise to the homogenization of American foods, reducing the diversity of tastes and textures considered acceptable by the public. With natural habitats quickly disappearing and being replaced by farmlands and towns, the populations of

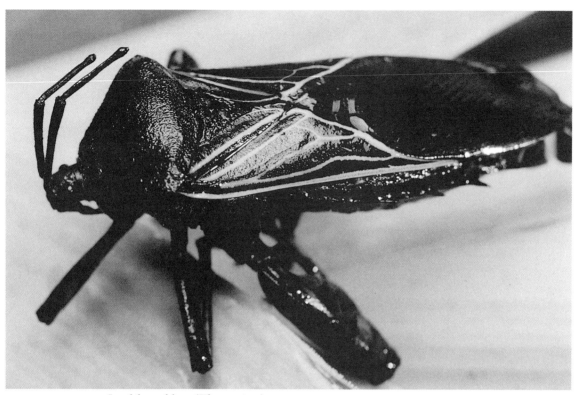
Leaf-footed bug (*Thasus gigas*)

many wild animals decreased, making them even less available as food and, in time, significantly modifying the character of the typical North American diet.

With further agricultural mechanization also came increased emigration to the cities. In urban areas, common insects began to be viewed not as part of the greater ecological balance, but merely as bothersome. Flies, mosquitoes, bedbugs, and fleas bit and itched, and cockroaches were thought of as dirty, disgusting indicators of squalor.

INSECTICIDES

From the earliest times that human beings first began to plant and harvest, it is likely that we have employed some type of rustic methods of insect control (the ingestion of insects being one particularly direct method). But as the United States dependence on agriculture increased, the first synthetic insecticides were formulated to combat the perceived enemy, the most devastating—and non-biodegradable—of these insecticides being dichloro-diphenyl-trichloroethane, better known as DDT. This was the beginning of an effort to create an insect-free agricultural environment and accelerated the serious damage humans were causing to the environment.

As more and more synthetic insecticides were developed, these toxic substances were absorbed not only by the insects they targeted, but also by domestic animals, the very food source upon which human beings were dependent. Each year the amount of toxic insecticides being used increases, as does their concentration in not only our foods, but also our water supply, our air, and our soil. Overexposure to insecticides causes cancer, birth defects, nervous disorders, and other serious diseases in human beings. The use of these chemicals continues to rise as their effectiveness continues to decline. Yet pests of all kinds are destroying more crops as resistant strains of insects develop and previously insignificant pests become major crop destroyers now that their predators have been chemically eliminated.

A NEW PERSPECTIVE

Though it might seem otherwise, not everyone in the United States has always been opposed to entomophagy. In the twentieth century, a new boom of immigration hit the United States, but unlike earlier waves of immigration, the majority of these new immigrants were not from Europe but from the American tropics and semitropics, people of mixed Latin and Amerindian descent in whom the practice of eating bugs was deeply ingrained. In addition, views on entomophagy became increasingly altered with the influx of Asian immigrants into the United States. For these immigrants entomophagy was not only a natural dietary habit but also a culinary luxury. The Asian community brought with them a taste for insects as well as a sophisticated tradition of preparing and preserving them. Rather than finding entomophagy barbaric, these immigrants considered insect dishes gourmet, and such dishes were appreciated and served at the very finest tables.

Many people would argue that, like so many other things, the acceptance of entomophagy is simply a matter of fashion—of public perception. If so, then what current trends might be seen as contributing to the increasing popularity of the practice of eating insects in the United States?

Certainly this increased visibility can be attributed partly to the similar rise in popularity of the science of insect study itself (entomology). Many universities in the United States and all over the world are offering more courses with an entomological basis and accepting dissertations on related themes. In my own teaching, I have formulated courses on entomophagy, as well as others on medicinal insects and insect recyclers, that have been used in Mexico, Peru, and China. There also have been expositions featuring insects—including edible ones—at the Natural History Museum in Los Angeles, at NASA, at the San Francisco Zoo, and at the Annual Fair of Edible Insects at the Montreal Insectarium in Quebec.

Currently, in some elementary and high schools in the United States, special-event days have been established on which students participate in excursions to capture and cook insects. Extremely popular, activities such as this have resulted in greatly elevating young people's awareness of how insects are used for food in other countries and the potential for increasing their use in more of them. As mentioned earlier, in some circles the practice of dining on insects has become very chic. With the never-ending quest for more unusual lifestyles—and more exotic foods—insects are presently finding themselves in vogue.

A good deal of the current interest in edible bugs can be attributed to American entomologist Gene DeFoliart, a professor emeritus at the University of Wisconsin at Madison. Dr. DeFoliart founded the *Food Insects Newsletter*, the first publication in the world to publish the work of formal and amateur researchers in the field of entomophagy. Through the publication of the *Food Insects Newsletter*, the how's, where's, and why's of insect consumption have begun to enjoy broader exposure and acceptance. A shelfful of books—Ronald Taylor's *Butterflies in My Stomach*, his and coauthor Barbara Carter's *Entertaining with Insects*, Berenbaum's *Bugs in the System* and *Dreamful Delicacies*, Patricia Quintana's *Mexican Foods*, and Diana Kennedy's *The Mexican Kitchen*—all have helped spread the word that insects make good food.

It is interesting to note that restaurants specializing in edible insects have begun to spring up across the United States. In Washington, D.C., a restaurant called The Insect Club began adding a selection of edible insects to its menu in 1994. Mark Nevin, the former chef at the Insect Club, said he bought 25,000 crickets and 25,000 larvae of mealworms each day for processing in the restaurant. Chefs in a number of American restaurants that include insects in their menus complain that they do not have a sufficient supply of insects to satisfy their demand. I personally have received requests for 300 kilograms of ants for a restaurant in Chicago, 500 kilograms for a restaurant in Los Angeles, and 400 kilograms for various restaurants in Cancun, Mexico. In 1992 the Explorer's Club in New York City held the celebratory dinner for the 100th anniversary of the New York Entomological Society featuring a menu composed of many insect dishes. Listed at the end of this chapter is the menu from the New York Entomological Society's banquet, followed by a modified version of the menu as it was recreated for Japanese television.

So cast aside the idea that insects are a food source for only underdeveloped countries. The time has come to lay down our misconception of insects as an inferior food and to keep pace with the rest of humanity, appropriately valuing what resources the planet offers. It is time to take a creative approach to entomophagy, to limit the use of dangerous pesticides and preservatives, and to explore the world of insects in ways we never dreamed.

New York Entomological Society
Centennial Banquet
May 20, 1992

At the Bar
Crudité with Peppery Delight Mealworm Dip
Spiced Crickets and Assorted Worms

Butlered Hors d'Oeuvres
Waxworm and Mealworm and Avocado California Roll
with Tamari Dipping Sauce
Wild Mushrooms in Mealworm Flour Pastry
Cricket and Vegetable Tempura
Mealworm Balls in Zesty Tomato Sauce
Mini Bruschetta with Mealworm Ganoush
Worm and Corn Fritters with Plum Dipping Sauce

Buffet
Chicken Normandy with Calvados Sauce
Rice Pilaf
Roast Beef with Gravy
Roasted Potatoes
Mediterranean Pasta
Melange of Vegetable Ragu
Mesclun Salad with Balsamic Vinaigrette
Assorted Seasoned Breads and Cricket Breads and Butter

Dessert Buffet
Lemon Squares
Chocolate Cricket Torte
Mini Cannoli
Peach Clafouti
Cricket and Mealworm Sugar Cookies
Coffee and Tea

Re-creation of
Banquet for Japanese TV
August 8, 1993

Stationary Hors d'Oeuvres
Spiced Roasted Trail Mix

Butlered Hors d'Oeuvres
Vegetable and Cricket Tempura with Apricot Dipping Sauce
Mealworm Fritters with Tomato Chutney
Mealworm Nori Balls with Ginger Soy Dipping Sauce

First Course
Steamed Banana Leaves with Mealworms and Soba Noodles
Garlic Fried Crickets over Pasta
Hearty Mixed Green Salad with Insect Croutons

Main Course
Paella with Thai Waterbugs, Shrimp, Clams, and Vegetables
Australian Kurrajong Grubs, Roasted New Potatoes and Gingered Carrots
Trio of Insect and Vegetable Tortillas with Black Beans and Rice
Fire Roasted Tarantula (sans abdomen)
All Served with Fresh Baked Cricket Bread

Desserts
Cricket Chocolate Torte with Candied Crickets, Fresh Chantilly Cream
Cricket Pie with Vanilla Ice Cream
Watermelon and Waxworm Sorbet
Coffee Service

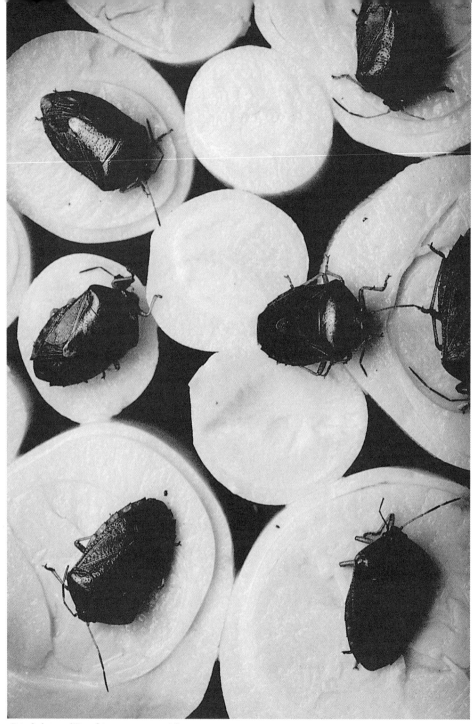

CHAPTER 4

Nutrition and Entomophagy

Stink bugs (*Euschistus taxcoensis*)

Necessary Nutrients

The majority of people living in industrialized nations have diets that are high in fat but deficient in many of the vitamins and minerals necessary for maintaining a healthy body. In direct contrast, populations in developing nations often suffer from a lack of fat intake and, because so few sources of these nutrients are available, from a severe lack of protein. Protein-packed, often high in fat, full of vitamins and minerals, and plentiful, insects can go a long way toward filling developing nations' nutritional needs.

In very simple terms, nutrition can be described as the relationship between food and our bodies and how the intake and the processing of food is essential to the body's maintenance, growth, and reproduction. Using protein, fat, carbohydrates, vitamins, and minerals (the essential nutrients), the body makes thousands more substances that are necessary for maintaining our physical well-being.

Below is a brief overview of the essential nutrients and the role they play in the health of our bodies.

Proteins. To our knowledge, no life-forms exist without proteins. Proteins are organic compounds made up of amino acids and are the primary structures of the human body. Not counting water, roughly one-half of a person's body weight is protein. A person's total protein is distributed throughout the body in the following way: muscles (33%), bone and cartilage (20%), skin (10%), and blood, body fluids, and tissue (37%). We build the protein we need for tissue repair and growth from the foods we eat, mainly from protein-rich animal food sources (beef, chicken, fish, pork and, in many parts of the world, insects) that supply complete proteins (those proteins having adequate amounts of the nine essential amino acids). Proteins from plants must be combined with one another to get the proper combination of the necessary amino acids.

Vitamins and Minerals. Vitamins and minerals have specialized roles in maintaining proper health. Vitamins A, C, D, E, and the B-complex vitamins are important for metabolizing carbohydrates, in the formation of collagen, and for building healthy skin and strong bones.

Minerals such as calcium, iodine, and iron are an essential part of all cells and body fluids, as well as being active in digestion, reproduction, brain activity, and all aspects of metabolism. Vegetarian diets are often deficient in certain nutrients because meat contains many of the vitamins and minerals needed by humans. As a result, vegetarians must pay careful attention to their diets to make sure they get an adequate supply of vitamins and minerals.

Fats and Carbohydrates. A highly concentrated source of energy, fats play an important role in conserving heat, forming certain hormones, and carrying vitamins A, D, E, and K to all the cells of the body. Fat contains twice the calories of other nutrients and is highly digestible. Our bodies require at least one tablespoon of fat per day—though North Americans consume an average of eight!

Carbohydrates are our primary fuel source provided by foods and most of us consume 200 to 300 grams of carbohydrates per day. Carbohydrates are broken down into two groups—sugars and starches—and are commonly found in grains, fruits, and vegetables. (For more information on human nutritional requirements see Table 5.)

How, you might ask, do insects as food fit into this nutrition profile? The answers might surprise you.

GOOD GRUB

Nearly two hundred years ago, English economist Thomas Malthus theorized that population would increase at a greater rate than food resources, and, despite the double-edged population controls of war and disease, this population explosion has indeed taken place. Population growth can be largely attributed to the many medical and technological advances in the last century, resulting in a greatly lowered infant mortality rate and an increased human life span. As the population continues to increase and dire food shortages become common, proper nourishment of the human race becomes a more pressing problem. Could the increased use of insects as food be the answer?

The diets of different ethnic groups and people of varying social levels are diverse, but nutritionists who have studied dietary practices most often promote the idea that an ideal diet is one that is low in fat and provides the necessary amounts of proteins, carbohydrates, vitamins, and minerals. One might expect that western countries, where the standard of living is high, would have more nutritious diets, but this is often not the case. Scientific knowledge and technological advancements have not always led to better nutrition. An example of this is the United States where individuals consume an average of 145 pounds of sugar and 60–65 pounds of fat per person annually.

As mentioned earlier, the most serious worldwide nutrient deficiency in human beings is that of protein, especially in people from developing countries.

TABLE 3

Amino Acid Content of Some Edible Insects (g/100g)

Essential Amino Acids	Water boatmen and Backswimmer eggs	Water boatmen	Grasshoppers (S. histrio)	Grasshoppers (S. purpurascens)
Isoleucine	2.9	2.9	5.3	4.2
Leucine	5.3	4.5	8.7	8.9
Lysine	3.8	2.8	5.7	5.7
Methionine	2.7	0.1	2.0	2.5
Cysteine	0.1	0.3	1.3	1.8
Total of sulphur amino acid*	2.8	0.4	3.3	4.3
Phenylalanine	2.7	2.4	11.7	10.3
Tyrosine	7.3	5.0	7.3	6.3
Total of aromatic amino acids**	10.0	7.4	19.0	16.6
Threonine	4.0	2.6	4.0	3.1
Tryptophan	0.6	0.4	0.6	0.7
Valine	2.0	2.7	5.1	5.7
Histidine	1.9	1.5	1.9	2.2
Total of Essential Amino Acids	**36.1**	**25.6**	**53.6**	**51.3**
Nonessential Amino Acids				
Aspartic Acid	1.8	4.6	9.3	8.7
Serine	5.6	3.2	5.1	4.8
Glutamic acid	8.8	7.1	5.3	10.7
Proline	n.a.	n.a.	7.2	6.2
Glycine	3.8	3.7	5.3	6.8
Alanine	5.0	4.4	7.6	6.4
Arginine	3.9	3.4	6.6	6.0
Total of Nonessential Amino Acids	**28.9**	**46.4**	**44.6**	**49.6**

* methionine + cysteine   ** phenylalanine + tyrosine

	Agave Billbug	Black Witch Moth	Leafcutting Ant	Honey Bee	Wasp (*Brachygastra azteca*)	Paper Wasp	WHO RDA*** (preschoolers)	WHO RDA (adults)
	4.8	4.1	5.3	4.1	5.1	6.4	2.8	1.3
	7.8	6.9	8.0	6.6	8.5	11.5	6.6	1.9
	5.5	6.3	4.9	6.0	6.1	4.3	5.8	1.6
	2.0	2.3	3.4	2.5	1.4	2.1		
	2.2	2.1	1.5	0.9	1.6	1.7		
	4.2	4.4	4.9	3.4	3.0	3.8	2.5	1.7
	4.6	9.5	8.8	7.0	4.1	4.2		
	6.4	4.4	4.7	4.1	6.5	6.6	6.3	1.9
	11.0	13.9	13.5	11.1	10.6	10.8	7.4	2.4
	4.0	4.0	4.3	4.4	4.4	4.9	3.4	0.9
	0.8	0.4	0.6	0.7	0.7	0.3	1.1	0.5
	6.2	4.8	6.4	5.9	6.4	6.7	3.5	1.3
	1.5	2.8	2.5	3.3	2.8	2.2	1.9	1.6
	45.8	**47.6**	**50.4**	**45.5**	**47.6**	**51.5**		
	9.1	8.7	9.0	9.8	8.4	7.4		
	6.6	5.8	4.4	4.8	4.5	5.1		
	15.7	11.4	10.4	13.8	16.4	12.5		
	5.4	7.3	7.9	7.5	6.4	7.7		
	6.1	5.1	6.6	5.8	6.7	7.3		
	6.5	6.7	6.6	5.5	5.8	6.0		
	4.4	6.7	4.7	6.4	4.4	3.4		
	53.8	**51.7**	**49.6**	**53.6**	**52.6**	**49.4**		

*** World Health Organization Recommended Daily Allowances

In the United States an adequate intake of protein (estimated to be between 43 and 63 grams per day, depending on age, weight, and gender) is usually not a problem, but in much of Asia, Africa, and South America the lack of dietary protein often leads to a number of health problems. In these poorer parts of the world, infants and toddlers often suffer from kwashiorkor, a disease characterized by an unnaturally bloated stomach; other symptoms of kwashiorkor include brittle hair, diarrhea, and stunted growth. Another disease, marasmus, results from a lack of both protein and sufficient caloric intake, and as a result the body literally starves, becoming a pile of bones with dry, baggy skin and sunken eyes.

Most edible insects are composed of between 30 and 85% high-quality proteins which contain all the amino acids essential to the construction and repair of the body's tissue (see Tables 3 and 4). Because of this, insects represent a significant portion of protein intake for people in many parts of the world. In woodland areas of Zambia, caterpillars known as mopanie worms act as the most important source of animal protein consumed. In the Central African Republic, larvae of *Pseudanthera descrepans* provide 50 to 60% of the total protein intake among Aka and Babinga pygmies. Unfortunately, Western influence in so much of the world has caused entomophagy to lose its appeal for many cultures that might ordinarily eat insects. Sadly, people want to eat what they see on television.

A second dietary necessity often in short supply in developing nations is fat. Many species of insects are excellent sources of fat—fat which can later be transformed into much needed energy (see Table 6). Insect fats also tend to be unsaturated, as opposed to saturated fats which are a factor in coronary disease. Over a million Americans have heart attacks every year and more than half of these die as a result. Often the proliferation of coronary disease in the United States is attributed to the high percentage of saturated fats consumed by Americans. Insects are also a good source of iron, riboflavin, niacin, and other vitamins and minerals.

TABLE 4

Protein content of common insects on a dry weight basis

Common Name	Protein %
Leafhopper	56.22
Yellow mealworm beetle (larvae)	47.76
House fly	
(larvae)	54.17
(pupae)	61.54
Darner (larvae)	56.22
June beetle (larvae)	42.62
Agave billbug (larvae)	55.56
Honey bee	
(larvae)	41.68
(pupae)	49.30
Water boatmen and backswimmer eggs	63.80
Water boatmen (adults)	53.80
Stinkbug	44.10
Leafcutting ant	58.30
Paper wasp (pupae)	57.93
Red-legged locust	75.30
Corn earworm	41.98
White agave worm	30.28–51.00
Red agave worm	37.10–71.00
Treehopper	44.84–59.57

Some of the major benefits of using insects as food is that they are easily located, easily harvested, and—compared to other food sources—relatively inexpensive. They are also easy to prepare and preserve. They can simply be dried in the sun or on a griddle.

INSECT TOXICITY

Eating food insects poses little, if any, health risk for the majority of people, especially if they have no history of allergy to insects or other arthropods. Nonetheless, because sensitivity can be acquired with repeated exposure to an allergen, a measure of prudence is advisable. Individuals with known allergies to insects or arthropods should exercise caution. Because insects and shellfish are in the same phylum, people who have suffered allergic reactions to lobster, shrimp, crayfish, and other such foods should avoid eating insects.

It is also important to remember that not all insects are edible and that we cannot go around eating insects willy-nilly. A large enough number of edible insect species are available on the market so that ingesting inedible ones should not be a problem. Enjoy your insects, just know your facts before eating them.

LIVESTOCK AND INSECTS

Insects play a role in the diet of many groups of animals, terrestrial as well as aquatic. In domesticated animals such as cows and sheep, the most important—and most expensive—part of their nourishment is supplying adequate protein. When fed with insects rather than conventional diets of corn and soybean supplemented with methionine, chickens, pigs, and fish grew better and had other improved organoleptic characteristics as a result of this change in diet. Trout fed with fly pupae and grasshoppers developed a superior color and taste.

TABLE 5

Recommended Daily Allowances

	Calories	Protein (g)	Fat (g)	Calcium (mg)	Phosphorus (mg)	Iron (mg)	Thiamin (mg)	Riboflavin (mg)	Niacin (mg)
Adult Male	2700	56	83	800	800	10	1.4	1.6	18
Adult Female	2000	44	67	800	800	18	1.0	1.2	13
Children (7–10)	2400	34	80	800	800	10	1.2	1.4	16
Infant (6 mos.– 1 year)	lbs x 47.7	lbs x 0.9	—	540	360	15	0.5	0.6	8

TABLE 6

Nutritional Values of Various Insects and Foods per 100 grams

Insect	Calories	Protein	Fat	Carbohydrates
June Beetle	77.8	13.4	1.4	2.9
Giant Water Bug	62.3	19.8	8.3	2.1
Red Ant	98.7	13.9	3.5	2.9
Red Ant Eggs	82.8	7.0	3.2	6.5
Silk Worm Pupae	98.0	9.6	5.6	2.3
Dung Beetle	108.3	17.2	4.3	0.2
Cricket	121.5	12.9	5.5	5.1
Short-tailed Cricket	112.9	12.8	5.7	2.6
True Water Beetle	149.1	21.0	7.1	0.3
Small Grasshopper	152.9	20.6	6.1	3.9
Large Grasshopper	95.7	14.3	3.3	2.2
Eggs	150	12	10	2
Pinto Beans	147	8.3	0.6	27.2
Lowfat Milk (2%)	49.2	3.3	2.0	4.9
Pasta (enriched, cooked)	125	4.4	1.3	23.1
Salmon (baked)	164.7	24.7	5.9	—
Ground Beef	288.2	23.5	21.2	—
Roasted Chicken	162.8	31.4	3.5	—
Pizza	241.7	12.5	7.5	32.5

Calcium	Phosphorous	Iron	Thiamin	Riboflavin	Niacin
22.6	207.0	6.0	0.29	1.19	3.99
43.5	225.5	13.6	0.09	1.50	3.90
47.8	206.0	5.7	0.24	0.88	3.38
8.4	113.4	4.1	0.15	0.19	0.92
41.7	155.4	1.8	0.12	1.05	0.86
30.9	157.9	7.7	0.19	1.09	3.44
75.8	185.3	9.5	0.36	1.91	3.10
88.2	163.4	14.4	0.26	1.78	2.31
36.7	204.8	6.4	0.31	3.51	6.85
35.2	238.4	5.0	0.23	1.86	4.64
27.5	150.2	3.0	0.19	0.57	6.67
50	178	1.4	0.06	0.50	—
47.8	164.4	3.0	0.18	0.09	0.39
121.7	95.1	—	0.04	0.16	0.08
10.0	58.8	1.6	0.14	0.08	1.19
30.6	316.5	0.6	0.21	0.16	5.8
10.6	169.4	2.5	0.04	0.19	4.4
15.1	227.9	1.0	0.07	0.12	13.72
182.6	179.3	1.33	0.28	0.24	3.48

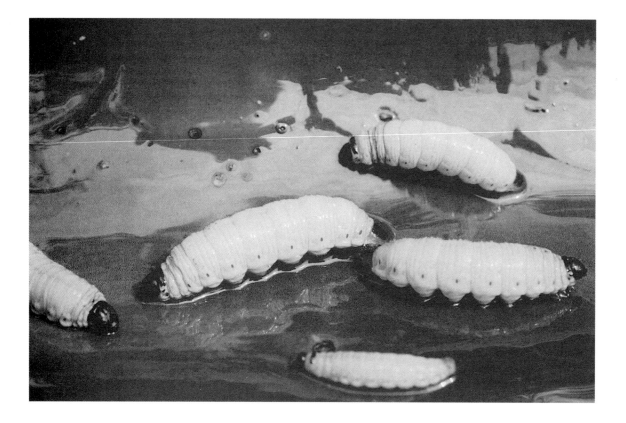

As can be seen in Table 6, the amount of protein found in water beetles and grasshoppers is nearly the same as that of such "high protein" foods as salmon and ground beef. The percentage of proteins and other nutrients in insects is very high (generally more than 50% of each gram), and their quality and digestibility is excellent. Compared with vegetable products (corn, wheat, beans, lentils, soybeans, etc.) or animal sources (beef, chicken, fish, etc.) the quantity of energy supplied by edible insects such as ants is actually quite large. Insects reproduce quickly and their complete biomass is usable, compared to fish of which 40% is waste. Another advantage in using insects as food is that they are cold-blooded and do not require energy to maintain the temperature of their body. This allows them to be more efficient in the conversion and transduction of energy and easier to raise than many other traditional foods. In economic terms, much money could be saved if we relied more on insects for our food supply and less on high-maintenance meat sources.

A LAST WORD

Before humankind can fully take advantage of insects as food, Western countries like the United States must lay to rest false perceptions of insects as unhealthy animals and realize that proper methods of selection and preparation can practically eliminate any health concerns we have regarding eating edible insects. As a species that mimics, we human beings tend to adopt the philosophies and beliefs of those around us, but, despite the excellent nutritional benefits, and because of this inaccurate and ignorant view, the practice and technological development of entomophagy as a means of preventing much world hunger is too often ignored.

PREPARING AND CLEANING INSECTS

Although it might seem unthinkable to suggest not washing your insects before you eat them, that is what I recommend. The pheromones of insects, which are responsible for a significant amount of their smell and taste, are lost when insects are washed. Of course, insects are still delicious if washed and prepared with condiments (for an alternate flavor), but their original, unique taste certainly will be diminished. Insects manufacture antibiotic substances in their exoskeleton that do not allow for the existence of any dangerous microorganisms, and during the frying process any germs will be killed with a cooking heat above 410° Fahrenheit. So leave the insects as they are—and if a you find a leaf or a speck of dirt that needs to be removed, do so with your fingers!

In general it is recommended that all herbivore insects not raised in a controlled cultivation—this includes grasshoppers and locusts—should not be fed for 4–12 hours before they are used. In the wild, insects may feed on bitter plants, which sometimes gives them an unpleasant taste, so it best to allow them the time to eliminate the contents of their digestive systems.

Once your insects are ready to use, place them in a plastic bag, then put them in the refrigerator for 15 minutes. This is especially recommended for mobile insects like grasshoppers (the cold slows them down). Choose the biggest, healthiest, darkest ones available and sort them according to the dish in which they'll be used, as well as according to how they'll be used—dried and ground, as a salad dish, or as a main dish. Avoid freezing insects, because freezing them reduces their taste. For best results, process your insects as soon as possible after they are harvested.

The most important thing to remember in preparing insects is that if any have died, these should be separated from the rest and thrown away. After doing this, weigh the remaining insects to ensure that you have the amount specified by the recipe. You may, of course, want to add your own personal touches here and there, varying the quantities used to correspond to your tastes.

With some species that are consumed at the insect's adult stage, you may choose to remove the wings and legs. While these may be eaten safely, some people prefer not to eat an insect's more prickly parts. For best results, these steps should be taken after all the other ingredients have been prepared so that the insects will be fresh.

If you are using canned or packaged insects, the quality control is assured and you may use them as instructed on the package; however, if they are purchased in a store or on the street, make sure they have been harvested from an area that does not use pesticides. You also can be adventurous and collect your own. Buy yourself a net for collecting grasshoppers, stink bugs, cicadas, treehoppers, beetles, and leafhoppers. For those insects with stingers—which can be dangerous for those people who are allergic—it is important to remember that insects are regulated by environmental temperature, so if you're harvesting them yourself the best way to avoid being stung is to collect them from their nests early in the morning or at dusk.

For a diverse number of species you can even cultivate your own insects by using cooked or raw kitchen wastes as food. This process requires several small plastic boxes of 50 cm x 25 cm x 15 cm (depending upon the quantity desired).

Place one or various pairs of insects in a box to allow them to reproduce. Depending on the species, reproduction will take from 45–90 days. On a regular basis you should replenish the organic wastes (the insects' food source), clean the excrement from the container, and give them water. You may want to cover the box with cheesecloth, securing the cloth around the top of the container with a rubber band. During this time the box should be periodically inverted into a sieve, so as to collect the insects at various stages of development, as well as to clean the excrement (which, incidentally, can be used in the garden as fertilizer). In this way all waste is recycled, and fresh, clean insects are yours for the eating.

¡Buen provecho!

Stink Bug Paté
(p. 76)

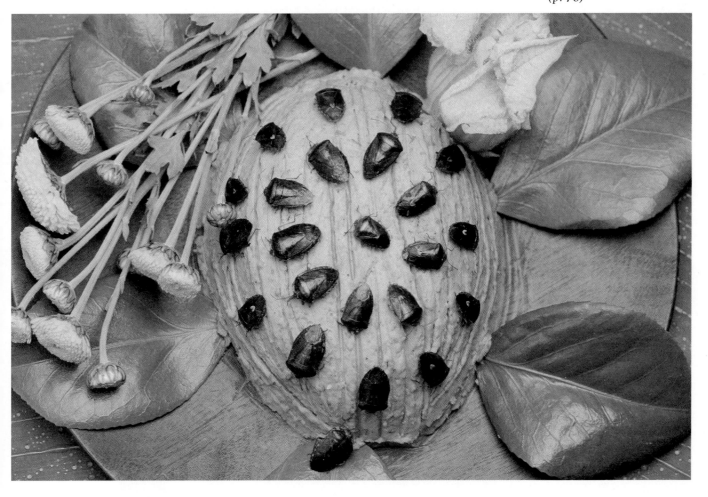

Ahuautle Amona
(p. 77)

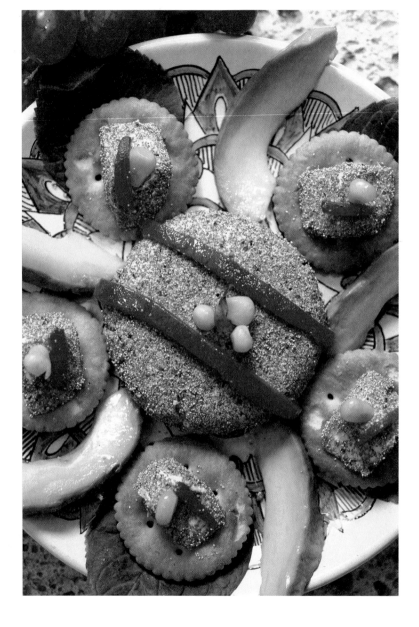

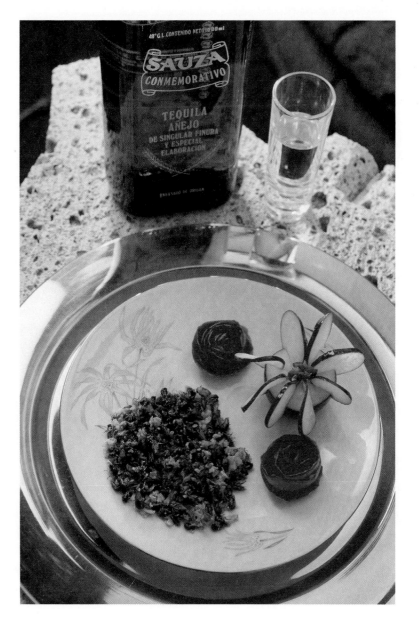

Periquitos Fritos
(*p. 78*)

Periquitos Fritos, close-up
(p. 78)

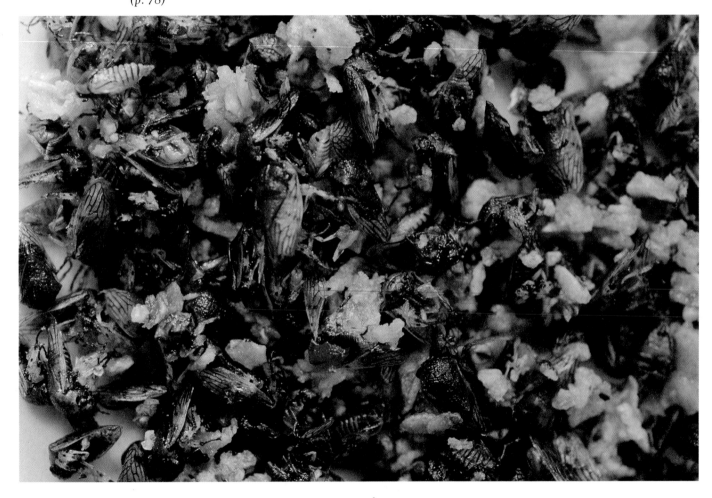

Black Witches a la Mediterraneo
(p. 79)

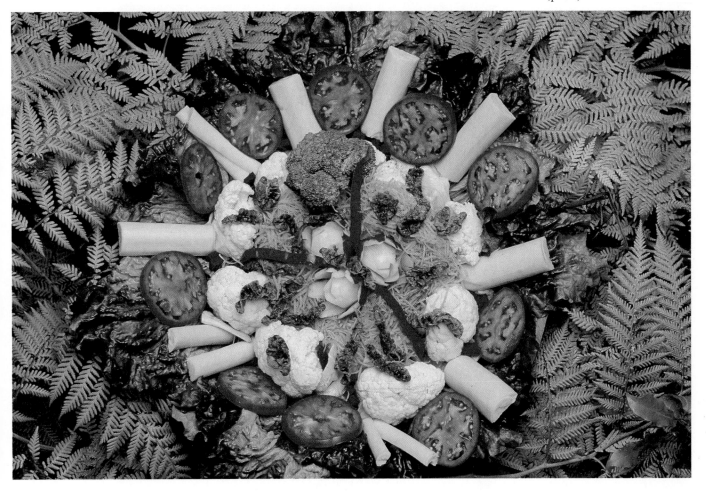

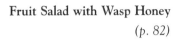
Fruit Salad with Wasp Honey
(p. 82)

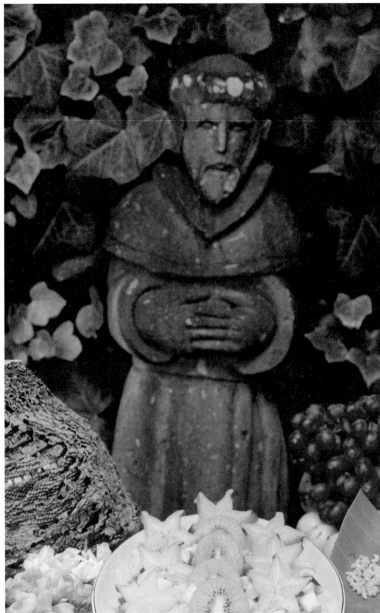

Mealworm Spaghetti
(p. 87)

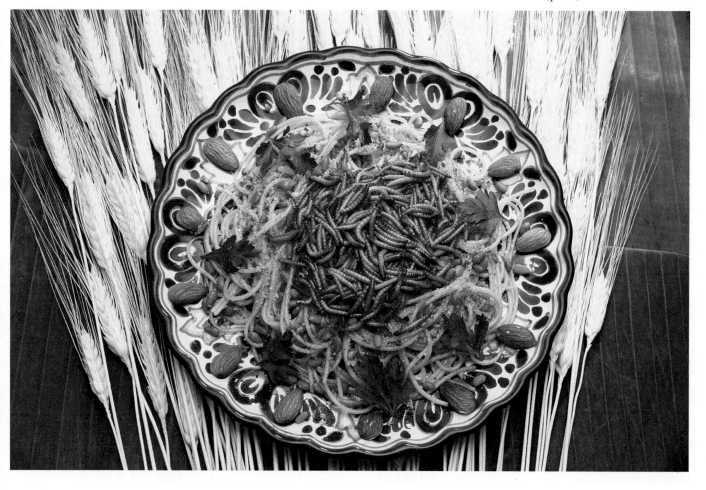

Mecapale Tamales
(p. 88)

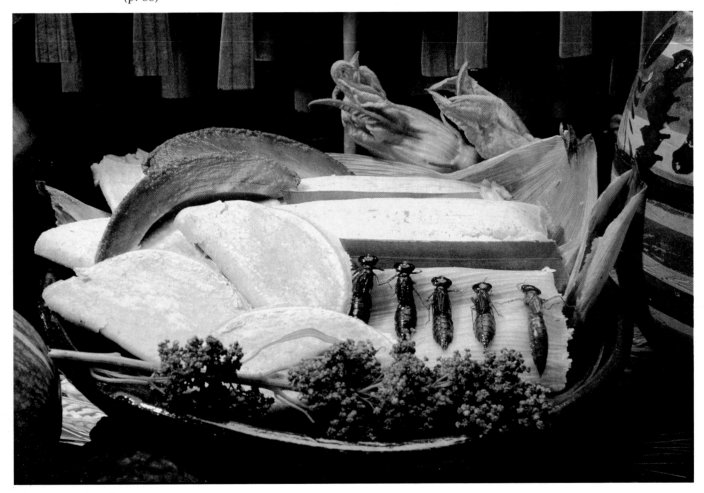

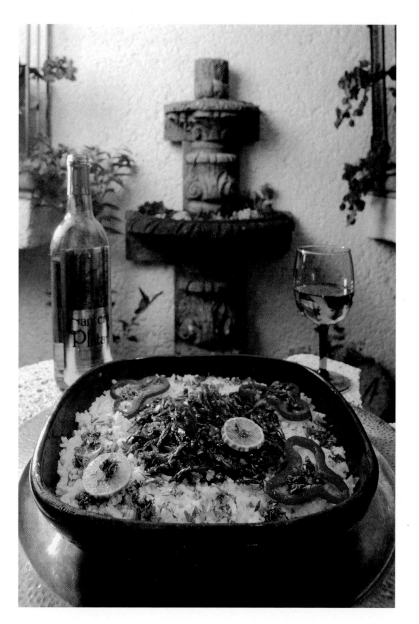

Crickets a la Papouasie
(p. 93)

Mango–Grasshopper Chutney
(p. 100)

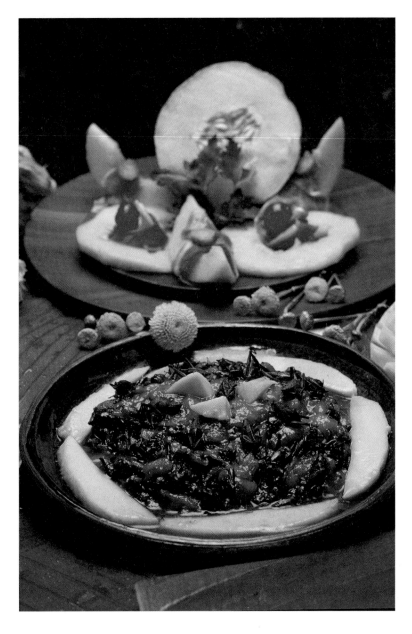

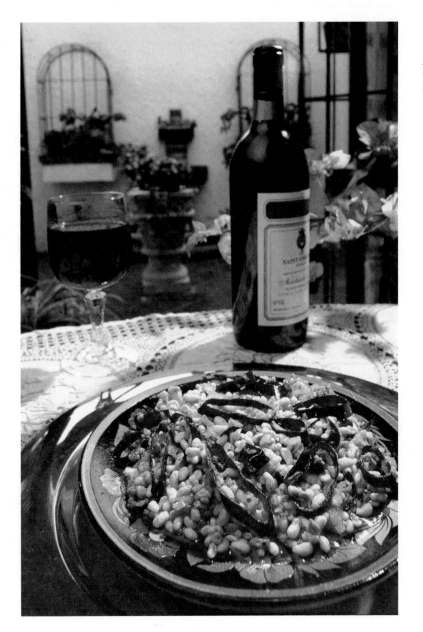

Escamoles al Guajillo
(p. 110)

Thai Brochettes
(p. 113)

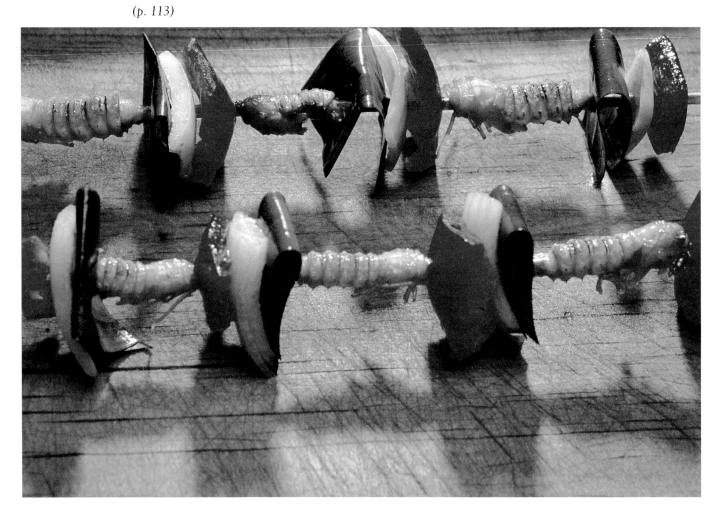

White Agave Worms in White Wine
(*p. 115*)

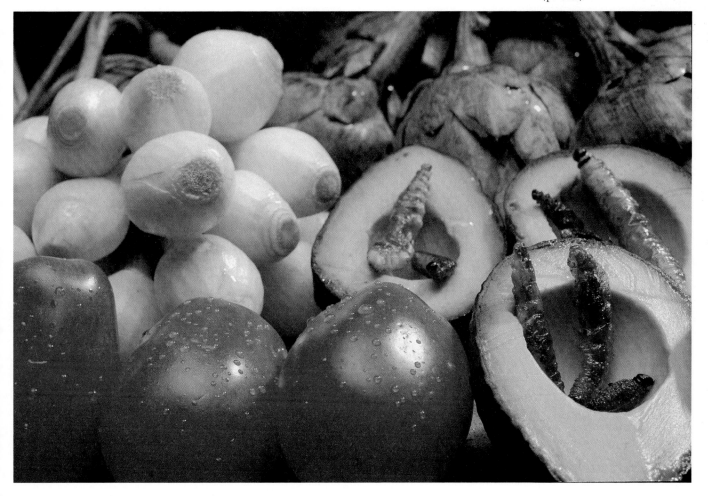

Pork Loin with Honey of the Virgin
(p. 117)

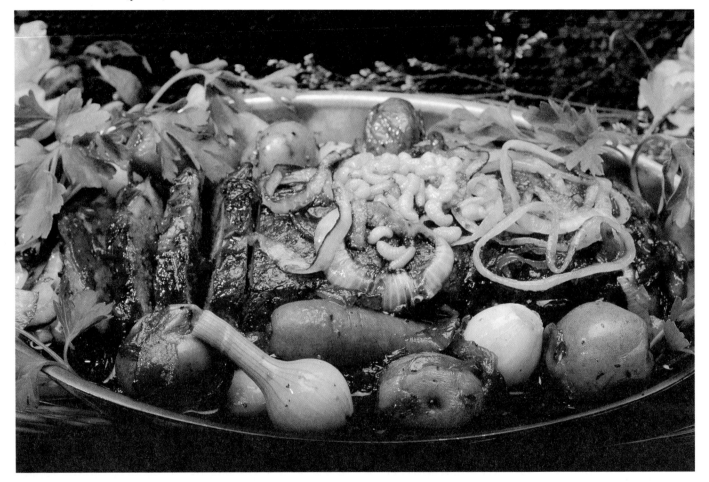

Leaf-Footed Bug Pizza
(p. 118)

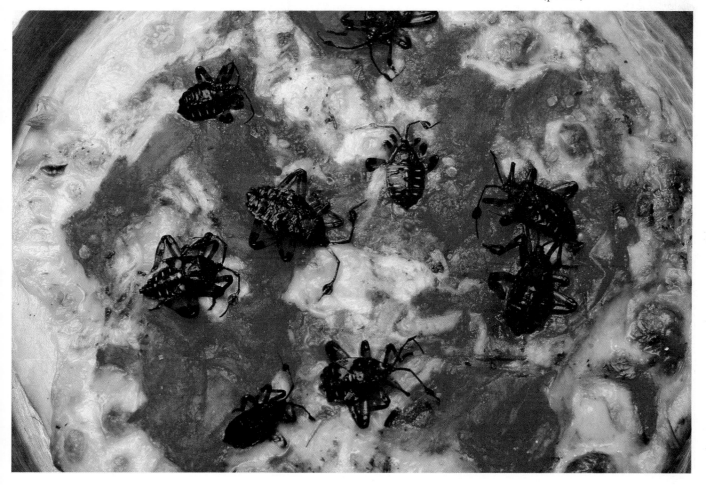

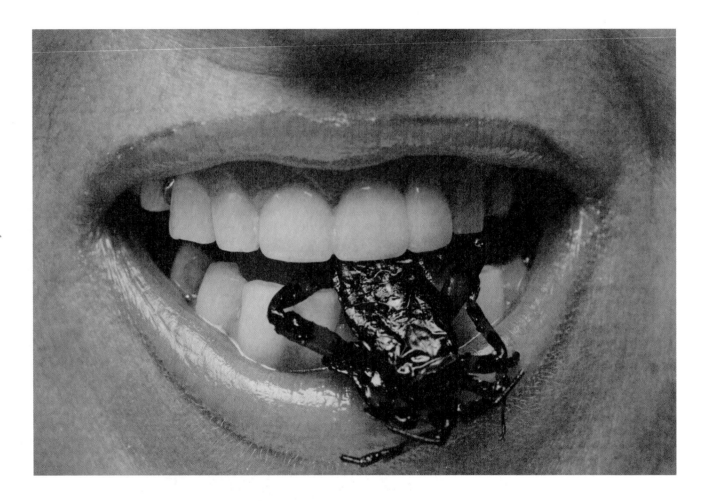

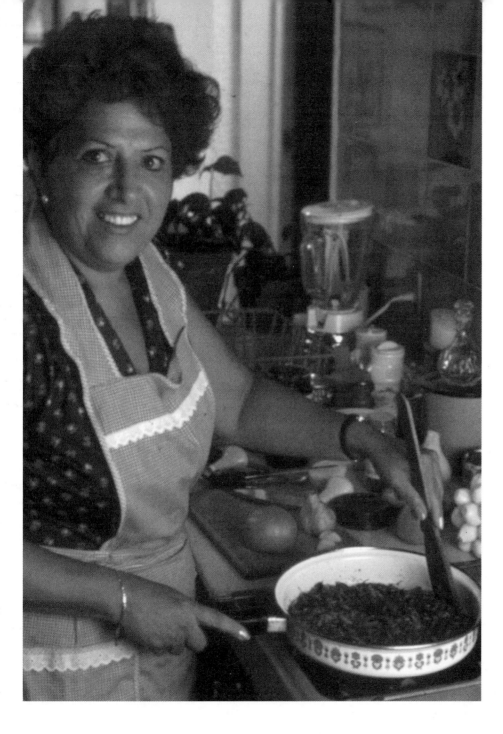

RECIPES

Appetizers

Acachapoli Cocktail

"Acachapoli" is the word for grasshopper in Nahuatl, the language spoken by the indigenous peoples of central Mexico, the inspiration for many of my recipes. This variation on shrimp cocktail uses grasshoppers, which, like their distant cousins, turn a bright, appetizing red when boiled.

$^1/_2$ **pound grasshoppers**
Juice of 2 lemons
Salt, to taste
$^1/_2$ **teaspoon chopped pequín chilies**
Pepper (optional)

Boil the grasshoppers in salted water. They will turn red when cooked. Drain and place on a griddle over low heat (or on a baking sheet in the oven) until dry.

Remove from heat, place in a serving dish, and squeeze lemon juice over them. Sprinkle with salt and pequín chilies. (The grasshoppers can also be steamed, and simply sprinkled with salt and pepper, to taste.) A delicious and nutritious appetizer which will impress and delight your guests.

Mexican Caviar

One of the most common insect foods in rural Mexico is ahuautle, the eggs of several different species of water boatmen and backswimmers that live together in lakes.

$^1/_4$ pound cream cheese or butter, or combination
$^1/_3$ pound *ahuautle*
1 small jar red peppers, or pimentos
1 egg, hard-boiled, finely chopped
1 package salted crackers

The ahuautle is enjoyed much like fine caviar: Spread cream cheese or butter on salted crackers, top with a dollop of the insect eggs, and garnish with a strip of red pepper. Sprinkle with the chopped hard-boiled egg. This is an exquisite, sophisticated, and novel appetizer. Surprise your guests!

Grilled Black Witches

Black witch moths are one of many species of butterfly and moth having suc-culent larvae. The larvae of giant silkworm moths are also eaten in this manner.

$^1/_2$ pound black witch larvae, dried
Freshly squeezed lemon juice, to taste
Pequín chilies, to taste
Paprika, to taste
$^1/_8$ teaspoon salt

Grill the larvae over medium-high heat, sprinkle with lemon juice, chopped pequín chilies, paprika, and salt. Toss lightly to mix. Place on a plate and serve as an appetizer.

Chicatana Spread

This is a simple appetizer with a nutty taste. "Chicatana" is the Nahuatl name for Atta cephalotes, a Mexican leafcutting ant. You may substitute a regional ant if you do not have access to chicatanas.

2 tablespoons peanut oil or butter
$^1/_3$ pound ants
$^1/_2$ small can chilies, drained
$^1/_4$ pound cream cheese
$^1/_8$ teaspoon salt
Ground cloves, to taste

Place the oil or butter in a frying pan over low heat. Add the ants and fry.

Place ants in a blender or food processor and purée. Add the chilies, cream cheese, salt, and ground cloves, to taste. Mix together and place in a serving dish to refrigerate.

Serve chilled, to spread on crackers or bread.

Stink Bug Paté
Illustration, p. 55

Despite their name, stink bugs are actually one of the most delectable of insects. Here, they add a unique flavor to a traditional paté.

¹/₃ **pound roasted stink bugs**
10 chicken livers
4 cloves garlic
1 small onion

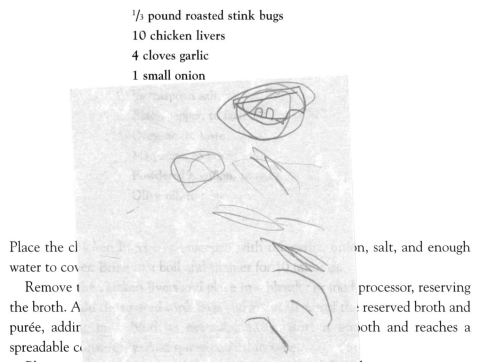

Place the ch... ...on, salt, and enough water to cov... ...boil ...simmer for...

Remove t... ...livers and place in a blender ...processor, reserving the broth. A... ...reserved broth and purée, addin... ...broth and reaches a spreadable c... ...

Place in a... ...with crusty french bread.

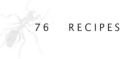

Ahuautle Amona

(Grandma's Waterboatmen Eggs)

Illustration, p. 56

$^1/_2$ pound cream cheese

$^1/_2$ cup sour cream

1 small can red peppers or pimentos

$^1/_8$ teaspoon salt

$^1/_4$ teaspoon pepper

A pinch of bouillon

Cumin, to taste

$^1/_3$ pound *ahuautle,* dried

Place all ingredients, except *ahuautle,* in a blender. Blend until smooth and thoroughly mixed. Place in a small bowl or other mold and chill until firm. To serve, release from bowl or mold, place on serving plate or platter, and gently spread with *ahuautle* to cover. Surround with rounds of pineapple centered with cocktail cherries. Serve with crackers.

Periquitos Fritos
(Fried Treehoppers)
Illustrations, pp. 57, 58

Periquitos, "little parrots," or "parakeets," is the common Spanish name for the oddly shaped insects known as treehoppers.

6 to 10 garlic cloves, minced
2 tablespoons peanut or olive oil
$^1/_2$ pound treehoppers
$^1/_8$ teaspoon salt
Pepper, to taste
2 plum tomatoes

Sauté the minced garlic in oil over low heat. Add treehoppers and fry. Add salt and pepper to taste.

Peel tomatoes, cut into strips and lay the peel in circles to form rosettes as a garnish. Quick, nutritious, and exquisite!

Salads

Black Witches a la Mediterraneo
Illustration, p. 59

Black witch moth larvae combine with traditional Mediterranean spices and vegetables in this tasty, nutritious salad ideal for sultry days, with a flavor similar to herring. Have your guests guess the ingredients. Won't they be surprised!

$^1/_2$ head lettuce, finely chopped

$^1/_3$ pound potatoes, cooked and cubed

$^1/_3$ pound carrots, cooked and cubed

$^1/_2$ pound peas, cooked

$^1/_2$ pound black witch larvae, dried

$^1/_2$ cup thyme vinegar

$^1/_2$ cup olive oil

Dill to taste

Ground coriander, to taste

$^3/_4$ cup parsley, minced

$^1/_8$ teaspoon salt, or more to taste

$^1/_8$ teaspon pepper, or more to taste

1 medium tomato, sliced (optional)

1 small onion (optional)

Avocado, peeled and sliced (optional)

Place the chopped lettuce in a bowl and add the potatoes, carrots, and peas.

Cut the larvae in pieces and fold into the potato-carrot mixture. Add the vinegar, olive oil, dill, coriander, parsley, and salt and pepper, to taste. If desired, slices of tomato, onion, and avocado may be added. Serve cold.

Rhodesia Salad

The peoples of central and southern Africa have some of the most established entomophagous cultures in the world. This salad is my adaptation of a dish you might find there.

$^1/_2$ head Romaine lettuce, finely sliced or chopped

$^1/_2$ cup olive oil

Juice of 1 lemon

1 teaspoon chopped dill

$^1/_8$ teaspoon salt

Pepper, to taste

2 tomatoes, cut in rounds

2 stalks celery, finely chopped

2 avocados, peeled and sliced

4 pears, sliced lengthwise

$^1/_2$ pineapple, sliced

$^1/_2$ pound roasted ant larvae or pupae

larvae or pupae to garnish (optional)

Place the chopped lettuce on a platter.

Whisk together the olive oil, lemon juice, dill, salt, and pepper and drizzle over the lettuce. Add the tomatoes, celery, avocado, pear, and pineapple. Sprinkle with the roasted, crunchy ant larvae and serve. (This dish can be nicely garnished with agave billbug larvae or larvae and/or pupae of bees or wasps.)

Wasp Salad

$^{1}/_{2}$ pound larvae and/or pupae of bees or wasps
$^{1}/_{2}$ cup olive oil
$^{1}/_{2}$ cup peanut oil
$^{1}/_{4}$ cup honey vinegar (or other vinegar)
$^{1}/_{2}$ pound mushrooms, finely chopped
$^{1}/_{4}$ head lettuce, finely chopped
1 can hearts of palm, chopped
1 mango, peeled and cut in pieces
1 teaspoon salt, or more to taste
$^{1}/_{8}$ teaspoon pepper, or more to taste

Fry the larvae in the olive oil at medium heat until they are crunchy. Place in a serving dish and add the peanut oil, honey vinegar, mushrooms, lettuce, hearts of palm, and mango. Mix well, adding salt and pepper to taste. This salad makes an excellent accompaniment to main course dishes.

Fruit Salad with Wasp Honey

Illustration, p. 60

Those who aren't ready to take the plunge and eat insects can still enjoy their products with this honeyed fruit salad. It may surprise some to learn that honey bees are not the only makers of honey; many bees and wasps produce delightful and unusual honeys. Those fortunate enough to have access to wasp honey should certainly use it; others can substitute the usual kind.

2 red apples, cut in wedges

2 golden apples, cut in wedges

3 peaches, cut in wedges

2 bananas, sliced

2 pears, diced

3 oranges, peeled and sectioned

3 mandarins, peeled and sectioned

2 kiwis, peeled and sliced

$^1/_8$ pound granola

$^1/_4$ cup raisins

4 ounces chopped macadamia nuts

1 cup wasp honey

$^2/_3$ cup whipped cream

Mix all the fruit together. Add the granola, raisins, nuts, wasp honey, and cream.

Padrecitos a la Anenez
(Dragonfly Seviche)

Padrecitos, "little fathers" in Spanish, are the larvae of dragonflies—acquatic larvae that live in ponds and slow streams and prey on mosquitoes and other insects. This modern variation on seviche works just like the shellfish version—the naiads are "cooked" by marinating them in lemon juice. Accompany the padrecitos with plenty of cold beer.

$^1/_2$ pound dragonfly larvae

lemon juice, enough to completely cover the larvae (approx.
   3 lemons)

1 small onion, diced

2 tomatoes, diced

$^1/_2$ handful parsley, chopped

$1^1/_2$ tablespoons olive oil

$1^1/_2$ tablespoons grapeseed oil

Thyme vinegar, to taste

Freshly minced dill, to taste

$^1/_8$ teaspoon salt

$^1/_8$ teaspoon pepper

2 avocados, peeled and sliced

Put the naiads, whole or in pieces, in lemon juice for three hours. Add the onion, tomato, parsley, vinegar, oil, dill, and the salt and pepper. Garnish with slices of avocado. Serve cold as a main course.

Soups

Cream of Asparagus Soup with Boll Weevil Croutons

$^1/_2$ pound boll weevil larvae, roasted

1 pound zucchini, diced

2$^1/_2$ cups chicken or vegetable broth

2 tablespoons butter

Salt, to taste

2 garlic cloves, minced

$^1/_4$ cup chopped onion

1 can condensed cream of asparagus soup

Pepper, to taste

Monterey jack cheese, grated

Sour cream, to taste

Place the larvae in a skillet and cook over medium heat until dry and crisp. Set aside.

Place the zucchini in salted water in a sauce pan and bring to a boil. Reduce heat and simmer over medium heat until soft. Add the garlic and onion and purée the zucchini along with the cooking water.

Melt the butter in a large soup pot and add the purée. Stir in the can of asparagus soup and the black pepper and cook for three minutes. Add the stock and cook a few minutes longer. Allow people to garnish their own soups with sour cream, cheese, and the roasted larvae.

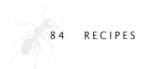

Metzolli Supreme

"Metzolli" is the Nahuatl word for the stem of the agave, where the larvae of the agave billbug can be found. Boll weevil larvae can be substituted.

$^1/_2$ pound agave billbug larvae, roasted

$4^1/_4$ cups chicken or beef broth

6 avocados, peeled and cut into pieces

1 cup cream

4 ounces cream cheese

$^1/_8$ teaspoon salt

$^1/_8$ teaspoon pepper

Place the larvae in a skillet and cook over medium heat until dry and crisp. In a soup pot, heat the broth to boiling. In a separate mixing bowl, mash the avocado and mix in the cream and cream cheese until well blended. Whip until fluffy. Stir whipped mixture into boiling broth. Lower heat and simmer for 3 minutes. Serve hot, garnished with roasted larvae to give this dish its singular flavor.

Main Courses

Baganda Rice

A delightful alternative to traditional fried rice! Red agave worms are the larvae you find in bottles of mescal and tequila. Corn earworms make a good substitute.

$^{1}/_{2}$ pound red agave worms

1 cup rice

2 cups water

1 cup sunflower oil

5 garlic cloves, minced

1 medium or $^{1}/_{2}$ large onion, thinly sliced

1 teaspoon salt

3 teaspoons lemon juice

3 sprigs parsley, washed and minced

2 strips bacon

Soak the rice in very hot water for 15 minutes, without boiling. Drain, rinse with cool water, drain again, and shake the strainer to remove the water.

Heat the sunflower oil in a pan until hot. Add the drained rice and spread to "fry," turning gently. When the rice is slightly golden, add the garlic and onion and sauté. Add the salt and parsley. Stir in the lemon juice and add enough cold water to cover. Cover the pan. Bring to a boil, then lower the heat and simmer until all the water is absorbed. Turn off the heat.

Fry the bacon in a skillet until crisp. Remove and crumble, reserving the bacon fat. Fry the worms in the bacon fat until browned. Chop and serve over the rice with the crumbled bacon.

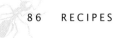

Mealworm Spaghetti
Illustration, p. 61

$^1/_2$ pound mealworms, roasted and diced

$4^1/_4$ cups water

1 tablespoon safflower oil

1 sprig marjoram

1 sprig thyme

2 bay leaves

$^1/_4$ onion

1 8-ounce package spaghetti

6–8 tablespoons butter

$^1/_4$ teaspoon salt

Olive oil, to taste

3–4 tablespoons finely chopped almonds

10 sprigs parsley

$^1/_2$ pound purple basil

$^1/_2$ pound ricotta cheese

Put the water in a pot and heat to boiling. Add the safflower oil, marjoram, thyme, bay leaves, and the onion. Bring to a boil and add spaghetti. Cook 20 minutes. Strain the spaghetti and herbs, and rinse with cold water.

Place the butter in a frying pan over low heat. Add the drained spaghetti, salt, and pepper. Finely chop the basil, parsley, and almonds and mix with the ricotta cheese and olive oil. Add to the spaghetti mixture and heat through. Top with the mealworms and serve.

Mecapale Tamales
Illustration, p. 62

"Mecapales" are the acquatic larvae of predacious diving beetles. They add an exotic touch to these traditional tamales. The acquatic larvae of dobsonflies, stoneflies, and damselflies are also used in Mexico.

8 ancho chilies (deveined)

5 black peppercorns, ground

2 tablespoons sunflower oil

4 garlic cloves, finely chopped

3 coriander seeds, crushed

2 cumin seeds, crushed

$1/8$ teaspoon dried thyme

1 sprig marjoram

Salt, to taste

Powdered bouillon, to taste

$3/5$ pound predacious diving beetle larvae

1 pound tomatoes (approx. 2 large)

$1/2$ pound lard

$2^1/4$ pounds *masa harina* (corn flour)

1 large handful plantain leaves (soaked in water ahead of time for half a day) or corn husks

To make the salsa:

Cook the tomatoes and chilies in boiling water for 2 minutes. Remove and pull the skins off. Mash together with the pepper and strain. Heat the sunflower oil in a frying pan and fry the mashed chile mixture in the oil. Add the garlic, coriander, cumin, thyme, marjoram, and the salt and bouillon and let rest for a while for the flavors to harmonize.

To make the tamales:

Heat the lard in a large pot over medium-high heat. Remove from heat and add the masa harina and salt to taste. Beat with a wooden spoon until dough reaches a smooth consistency. Drain the previously soaked plantain leaves and wipe with a clean, dry cloth. Spread the plantain leaves with a thin layer of dough, the chile mixture, and the larvae—in that order—on the concave part of the leaf. Fold the leaves lengthwise and horizontally and place seam-side down in a colander within a pot over 2 cups of water. Make layers of tamales and cover with the remaining leaves. Bring the water to a vigorous boil and steam for one hour, replenishing water as needed.

Ahuautle Omelette

Ahuautle—the eggs of water boatmen and backswimmers—combine beautifully with the kind of eggs we are more familiar with to make an exquisite breakfast dish with plenty of protein to start the day off right.

6 chicken eggs
1 small onion, finely chopped
2 serrano chilies, diced
$^1/_3$ pound *ahuautle*
3 tablespoons canola oil
salt, to taste

Put the chicken eggs in a bowl and use a fork to whisk in the onion, chilies, and ahuautle. Heat the oil in a frying pan. Add the egg mixture to the hot oil and cook until it has set all the way through. Fold, cut into triangles, sprinkle with salt to taste, and serve.

Teclates Omelette

"Teclates" are the brood of the reproductive caste of ants in the Nahuatl tongue. They add a delicious hint of nut to this herbed omelette.

5 eggs
1 tablespoon parsley, minced
$^1/_2$ tablespoon cilantro, minced
2 tablespoons onion, diced
1 tomato, finely chopped
Salt, to taste
Pepper, to taste
Ground coriander seed, to taste
2 tablespoons safflower oil
$^1/_5$ pound ant larvae, roasted
Slivered parmesan cheese (optional)
Red bell pepper, roasted and sliced (optional)

Whisk the eggs in a bowl, and mix in all the ingredients except the larvae, the oil, and the salt and pepper. Heat the oil in a frying pan, add the herbed vegetable–egg mixture, and cook until set. Place the larvae in the center, heat through, fold, and serve. Garnish with slivers of cheese and strips of roasted red pepper if desired.

Black Witch Fondue

$^1/_2$ pound black witch moth larvae, dried,
   or other butterfly or moth larvae
$1^1/_2$ cups swiss cheese, grated
$1^1/_2$ cups Monterey jack cheese, grated
$^1/_4$ cup Gruyere cheese, grated
1 cup white wine
$^1/_2$ cup Kirsch (cherry liquor)
1 loaf crusty bread, cubed

Heat the white wine and Kirsch in a fondue pot. Mix the cheeses together and add one handful at a time, stirring until melted. Chop the larvae and fold into the fondue. Serve the fondue along with cubed bread in a basket. Use individual fondue forks or skewers to dip the bread cubes into the fondue. Keep the cheese warm over low heat. Serve with white wine—a good Riesling is especially nice with this fondue!

Crickets a la Papouasie

Illustration, p. 63

These garlicky crickets are exquisite, with a superior flavor to shrimp. You will be delighted when you try them.

8 tablespoons butter
1 head garlic, cloves peeled
$1/2$ pound live crickets
$1/8$ teaspoon salt
Parsley, chopped, to taste
Powdered bouillon, to taste

The crickets should have one day of fasting so they will be cleansed internally. Mince the peeled garlic cloves. Place the butter in a frying pan and add the chopped garlic. When garlic is browned, add the crickets and salt and fry over low heat until crickets are slightly crunchy, approximately 3 minutes.

Sprinkle with chopped parsley and powdered bouillon and serve with white rice.

Cricket Croquettes

$^2/_3$ cup olive oil

$1^1/_4$ pound crickets

1 onion, diced

3 large peppercorns

1 pound fresh spinach, chopped

Salt and pepper, to taste

3 eggs

$^1/_2$ pound peeled potatoes, boiled and mashed

1 cup plus 2 teaspoons flour

8 tablespoons bread crumbs

1 cup safflower oil

To prepare the croquettes:

Heat the olive oil in a frying pan and sauté the crickets until crispy. Remove the crickets and drain on a paper towel. Place the onion in the same pan of oil and sauté until golden. Add the spinach, salt, and pepper and cook until liquid is evaporated. Combine spinach and crickets in a bowl and set aside.

In a blender, liquefy one onion and the peppercorns. To this mixture add 2 eggs, the mashed potatoes, salt, and pepper, and combine. Blend in 2 teaspoons flour.

Prepare for dredging: place a cup of flour on a plate, 1 beaten egg in a small bowl, and the bread crumbs in a shallow dish. For each croquette, take a small

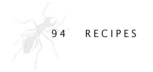

handful of the potato mixture, shape it into a ball in the palm of your hand, and poke a hole in one side. Stuff a small spoonful or healthy pinchful of the spinach-cricket mixture into the ball's center, and pinch the batter closed to contain the stuffing.

Heat the safflower oil in a skillet to the smoking point and reduce heat to low. Roll each croquette in flour, dip in beaten egg, and roll in the bread crumbs. Fry croquettes in heated oil, rolling with a wooden spatula until golden brown on all sides.

Salsa for Cricket Croquettes

1 onion, minced
1–2 tablespoons olive oil
2 medium tomatoes
$^1\!/_2$ teaspoon oregano
$^1\!/_3$ teaspoon marjoram
1 tablespoon honey vinegar
salt, to taste

To prepare the salsa:

Preheat oven to 450°F. Place tomatoes on a baking sheet, rolling them frequently, until their skins are blackened. Remove skins, mash, and strain.

Heat the oil in a frying pan and sauté the onion and roasted tomatoes. Add oregano and marjoram. Remove from heat and add honey vinegar and salt.

Grasshoppers en Papillote

Cooking en papillote (in parchment, or foil, envelopes) is a wonderful way to seal in all the flavors of your dish and get them to harmonize. It also makes for a very festive meal, with each guest opening their own "present" at the table—which with this dish can lead to some memorable moments!

$1/2$ pound mushrooms
1 tablespoon butter
3 garlic cloves, minced
Salt and pepper, to taste
$1/2$ cup white wine
1 tablespoon chopped parsley
1 pound grasshoppers
8 strips smoked bacon
8 pieces aluminum foil, each 1 foot square

Boil grasshoppers in salted water until they turn pink, approximately 10 minutes. Remove and set aside. Preheat oven to 300°F.

Clean the mushrooms and slice thinly. Heat half of the butter and sauté the mushrooms and the garlic for 10 minutes. Season with salt and pepper to taste. Add the wine and stir, sprinkle with parsley, and cook over low heat for 20 minutes.

Fry the grasshoppers until dry. Rub the remaining butter on one side of each piece of aluminum foil. Wrap the grasshoppers in the strips of bacon, add salt and pepper, and place on the buttered aluminum foil pieces. Divide the mushroom mixture among them and fold up the aluminum foil to seal tightly.

Place in the preheated oven and cook for 15 minutes. Serve still enclosed in the foil.

Acachapoli al Curry
(Curried Grasshoppers)

Spice up your menu, increase your cultural gastronomy, lose your prejudices—these curried grasshoppers are finger licking good!

$^1/_2$ cup peanut oil
$^1/_2$ small onion
1 clove garlic, peeled
$^1/_2$ pound grasshoppers
Ground anise, to taste
Ground cloves, to taste
Ground curry, to taste
Ground mustard, to taste
$^1/_8$ teaspoon salt
Ground pepper, to taste
Powdered bouillon, to taste

Boil the grasshoppers in 6$^1/_2$ cups of salted water until they turn pink, approximately 10 minutes. Spread on a paper towel and let dry.

Heat the peanut oil in a frying pan and sauté the onion and garlic over low heat until browned. Add the grasshoppers, the anise, cloves, curry, mustard, salt, pepper, and bouillon. Add some water and let it evaporate. Serve this curry treat hot on toast, in tacos, or with white rice. For heightened flavor, try adding young grasshoppers.

Pipian Chapoli
(Nutty Spiced Grasshoppers)

Pipian is a powder made from ground, toasted pumpkin seeds and other plants, and is traditional in Mexican cooking. If you cannot find it in a Latin American grocery store, it is easy to make your own. Epazote, a member of the goosefoot family, is a common Mexican herb. If you cannot find it substitute a combination of sage and oregano. The combination of these traditional ingredients with grasshoppers (in Nahuatl, "acachapoli") makes sumptuous soft tacos.

2 scallions, cut in pieces

$1/2$ pound tomatillos, cut in pieces

5 radish leaves

2 leaves epazote

5 serrano chilies

1 handful parsley

5 garlic cloves, mashed

3 tablespoons corn oil

1 tablespoon olive oil

$1/2$ cup pumpkin seeds, toasted and ground

$1/4$ cup sesame seeds, toasted and ground

3 cumin seeds, toasted

$1/2$ pound grasshoppers

$1/8$ teaspoon salt

1 cup bouillon

tortillas, for serving

Preheat the oven to 350°F. Place the grasshoppers on a baking sheet and roast for 10 minutes.

Place the scallions, tomatillos, radish leaves, epazote, serrano chilies, parsley, and garlic in a blender or food processor and liquefy.

Heat the combined oils in a frying pan. Add the ground pumpkin seeds and fry over medium heat, stirring to prevent burning. Add the ground sesame seeds and the toasted cumin seeds. Season with salt, mixing thoroughly.

Add the bouillon a little at a time, stirring, and cook until thickened. Add the roasted grasshoppers. Spoon the filling into the warmed tortillas and serve.

Mango–Grasshopper Chutney

Illustration, p. 64

$^1/_2$ pound grasshoppers

$^3/_4$ cup peanut oil

$^1/_4$ medium onion, minced

5 garlic cloves, minced

1 teaspoon curry powder

Pinch of ground cloves

$^1/_8$ teaspoon salt

Juice of 3 lemons

1 jar mango chutney

3 cumin seeds, ground

Boil the grasshoppers in salted water until they turn pink, approximately 10 minutes. Spread on a paper towel and let dry.

Heat the oil over low heat, add the onion and garlic, and sauté. Add the grasshoppers and fry until crisp. Sprinkle with the curry, cloves, and salt. Add the lemon juice, the cumin, and finally the mango chutney.

Water Boatmen Fritters

5 eggs
1 teaspoon salt
Black pepper, to taste
Bouillon, to taste
$^1/_3$ pound water boatmen, roasted
$^1/_2$ cup canola oil
Cooked artichokes, optional garnish

Seperate the egg whites from the yolks. Whip the egg whites until stiff peaks form. Add salt, pepper, and bouillon. Whisk in the egg yolks one at a time, beating continuously. Add the roasted water boatmen.

Heat the oil in a frying pan and drop spoonfuls of the egg mixture into the oil. Fry until water boatmen are browned. Place the fritters on a platter and surround with cooked artichokes dressed with butter and pepper. Enjoy the shrimp-like taste!

Giant Water Bug Eggs in Garlic

1 cup olive oil
1 head garlic, cloves peeled and minced
1 small or $^{1}/_{2}$ medium onion, minced
$^{1}/_{2}$ pound fresh giant water bug eggs
1 handful parsley, chopped
White pepper, to taste

Heat the oil in a frying pan. Sauté the garlic in the hot oil until golden. Add the minced onion and the water bug eggs and sauté until golden. Add the pepper and parsley and serve hot.

—

Water Boatmen Tortas

$^{1}/_{2}$ pound water boatmen, dried

1 small or $^{1}/_{2}$ medium onion, minced

4 garlic cloves, minced

1 tomato, seeds removed, finely chopped

2 epazote leaves, finely chopped

$^{1}/_{8}$ teaspoon salt

5 eggs

1 cup canola or olive oil

Bouillon, to taste

Pepper, to taste

Perkins sauce, to taste

Soy sauce, to taste

Seperate the egg whites from the yolks. Whip egg whites until stiff peaks form. Continue to beat, and whisk in the egg yolks, one at a time. Mix in the water boatmen, the onion, the tomato, and the epazote. Add the salt, pepper, bouillon, a trickle of Perkins sauce, and a trickle of soy sauce.

Heat oil in a frying pan. Add this mixture a spoonful at a time and fry. Remove fried tortas and cover each with salsa (see next page). Serve these delicious novelties on a platter.

Salsa for Water Boatmen Tortas

3 tomatoes
$^{1}/_{2}$ onion
1 garlic clove
$^{1}/_{8}$ teaspoon salt
1 sprig epazote, chopped
$^{1}/_{8}$ cup canola oil

Place all ingredients except the epazote and the oil in the blender and liquefy. Heat the canola oil in a frying pan and fry this mixture. Season with the epazote. Dress the tortas with the salsa.

Braised Ant Brood

$^1/_2$ pound ant larvae and pupae
1 stick butter
$^1/_8$ teaspoon pepper
$^1/_8$ teaspoon salt
Powdered anise, to taste
1 cup white wine

Melt the butter in a frying pan over low heat. Fry the larvae and pupae until they turn a white, opaque color, then add salt and pepper, the anise, and white wine. Serve with bread.

Chop Suey Ants

The nutty flavor of the fried ant larvae and pupae mix nicely with the flavors of the tofu, vegetables, and soy sauce to make a classic Oriental dish.

1/2 cup canola oil
1 cup cooked rice
1 pound ant larvae and pupae
2 tablespoons minced onion
3 tablespoons chopped jícama
1/2 cup diced carrots
1 tablespoon minced celery
2 tablespoons diced zuchini
1/2 cup diced tofu
1 egg, hard-boiled and finely chopped
1 egg, beaten
1/8 teaspoon salt or pepper
Soy sauce, to taste

Heat half the oil in a frying pan over medium heat. Add the rice and fry.

In a separate pan, heat the remaining oil and fry the onion, jícama, carrots, celery, zuchini, and tofu. When fried, add this vegetable mixture to the rice. Stir in the diced, cooked egg and then the raw, beaten egg, and mix thoroughly. Add the larvae and pupae, fry until sizzling, and sprinkle with salt and pepper. Serve in individual bowls and add soy sauce to taste.

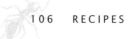

Escamoles al Pulque

Pulque is a Mexican alcoholic drink made from the fermented juice of the agave cactus. If you have no access to it try the recipe that follows this one instead.

$^1/_3$ **pound ant larvae and pupae**
2 cups pulque
dried fruits in syrup

Place the pulque and the ant larvae and pupae in a bowl and let marinate for one day. Roast until dry and serve with rounds of fresh tuna, peach, mango, or pineapple in syrup.

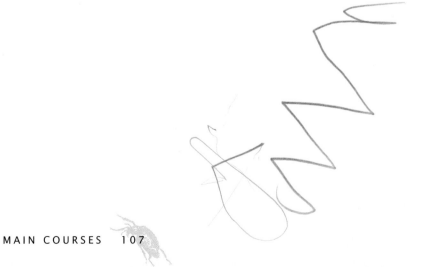

Ant Brood with Beer

3 bottles good beer
Aromatic herbs, as desired, to taste (bay leaves, oregano,
   thyme, marjoram)
1 pound ant larvae and pupae
Salt, to taste
Pepper, to taste

Place the beer and the aromatic herbs in a deep bowl, and allow to sit for two days at room temperature. Add the larvae and pupae and continue to marinate for one day. Serve with salt and pepper, to taste.

Accompany with toast spread with cream cheese. Delicious!

Escamoles a la Mexicana

(Ant Brood Tacos)

2 tablespoons butter or peanut oil
$^1/_2$ pound ant larvae and pupae
3 serrano chiles, raw, finely chopped
1 tomato, finely chopped
Pepper, to taste
Cumin, to taste
Oregano, to taste
1 handful cilantro, chopped
Taco shells, to serve

Heat the butter or oil in a frying pan and fry the larvae and pupae. Add the chopped onion, chilies, and tomato, and season with salt. Sprinkle with the ground pepper, cumin, and oregano, to taste.

Serve in tacos and garnish with cilantro.

Escamoles al Guajillo

(Spicy Ant Brood)

Illustration, p. 65

7 guajillo or other mild chilies

10 tomatillos

2 large tomatoes

8 garlic cloves

1 small onion

1 pound ant larvae and pupae, roasted or fried

2 tablespoons peanut oil

$1/8$ teaspoon salt

White pepper, to taste

Cumin, to taste

Powdered bouillon, to taste

Garnish, optional:

    sautéed onion rounds

    strips of guajillo chilies

    sprigs of sage

Drop the tomatoes into boiling water for 30 seconds. Remove them and pull off skins. Devein the chilies and toast them on a grill. Place in a pot with just enough water to cover and bring to a boil. Lower heat and simmer until soft. Add the tomatillos and cook. Put all this in a blender. Add the garlic, onion, and tomato and blend. Heat the oil in a skillet, add contents of blender, and cook. Add the pepper, salt, bouillon, and the roasted or fried ant larvae and pupae. Garnish with rounds of sautéed onion, strips of guajillo chilies, and sprigs of sage.

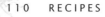

Mien Yao Beetles

In the Far East, which has taken entomophagy to culinary heights, water bugs are one of the most prized of foods. Here is my own version of a dish the typical traveller might stumble across while touring the region.

1/4 onion
3 tomatoes
2 tablespoons peanut oil
1/2 pound predacious diving beetle larvae
1 handful parsley
1 jicama, sliced in thin rounds
3 carrots, cut very fine
3 scallions, chopped
3 garlic cloves, minced
5 garlic greens, chopped (optional)
1/2 teaspoon powdered bouillon
1/2 cup water
Salt, to taste

Place the onion, garlic, and tomato in the blender and liquefy. Heat the oil in a skillet, add the blended mixture, and fry. When it is fried, add the larvae, parsley, jícama, carrots, scallions, and garlic greens and fry for 10 minutes. Season with salt and bouillon, add water, and cook until slightly thickened.

Batter-fried Dragonflies

5 eggs
$^1/_8$ teaspoon salt
$^1/_8$ teaspoon pepper
$^1/_3$ pound dragonfly larvae
2 tablespoons flour
1 cup canola oil
$^1/_2$ cup bread crumbs
Juice of 2 lemons

Separate the egg whites from the egg yolks. Set the yolks aside. Place the egg whites in a mixing bowl and whip until stiff peaks form. Whisk in the salt and pepper and egg yolks, one at a time, beating constantly.

Heat the oil in a frying pan. Dredge the rinsed larvae in flour, dip them in the beaten egg, roll in breadcrumbs, place in the hot oil and fry briefly. Add lemon juice and serve. This is a great way to prepare almost any edible insect.

Thai Brochettes
Illustration, p. 66

The larvae of various species of beetles that feed on the cellulose in tree trunks are a popular food with cultures around the world. As there are so many, I haven't specified a particular species in this recipe, though long-horned beetles, metallic wood-boring beetles, weevils, and bessbugs are all good North American choices.

1/3 pound salted peanuts (peeled and ground)
6 garlic cloves, minced
Ground cloves, to taste
Ground cardamom, to taste
1 cup coconut milk
1 tablespoon lime juice
2 tablespoons soy sauce
Salt, to taste
1 1/2 cups tree trunk beetle larvae
1 handful fresh lemongrass (cut in pieces)
1 onion, or more to taste, cut in chunks
Wooden skewers
Canned pineapple in syrup, cut into pieces, optional

To make the sauce, purée the peanuts, garlic, cloves, and cardamom with the coconut milk. Add the lime juice, soy sauce, and salt to taste, mixing thoroughly.

Cut the onion into pieces suitable for skewering (try cutting onion into quarters, then cutting each piece in half again.) For each skewer, put 6 to 10 beetle larvae on a stick, interspersing with pieces of lemongrass and onion dipped in the sauce. (Pieces of pineapple in syrup can also be added to the brochettes if desired.) Place prepared skewers on a grill for 5 minutes. Brush with the remaining sauce and continue to cook on the grill until sizzling, approximately 4 minutes.

White Agave Worms in White Wine

Illustration, p. 67

1 pound white agave worms
1 cup white wine
Salt, to taste

Harvest the worms in season and place in a soup pot with white wine (more or less worms may be prepared; the ratio is always 1 pound worms to 1 cup white wine). Bring to a boil for several minutes, remove from heat, and add a little salt to taste. Serve on avocados or other fresh fruits and vegetables.

Sago Soufflé

Sago are the larvae of a beetle found in palm trees in Southeast Asia and eaten by the locals. Since they are not available in North America, I have substituted the fat and succulent larvae of the agave billbug.

$^1/_2$ pound agave billbug larvae, roasted
6 potatoes, peeled and cooked
2 tablespoons butter
Milk, as needed
$^1/_8$ teaspoon salt
$^1/_8$ teaspoon pepper
6 eggs
1 tablespoon flour, sifted

Preheat oven to 300°F.

In a large mixing bowl, mash the potatoes with butter, milk, and salt and pepper. Stir in the roasted larvae.

Place the eggs in a separate bowl and whisk with a fork. Add the sifted flour to the eggs and mix both into the mashed potatoes.

Grease a baking mold with butter and fill with the potato mixture. Place in oven and bake for about 15 minutes. Turn out onto a platter and serve.

Pork Loin with Honey of the Virgin

Illustration, p. 68

In Mexico the delicate and much prized honey of stingless bees is known as "honey of the virgin." It is well worth seeking out, though this still makes a fine dish with regular honey.

2 pounds pork loin
Salt, to taste
Coarse black pepper, to taste
1 cup canola oil
Ground cinnamon, to taste
Ground cloves, to taste
Ground anise, to taste
Ground mustard, to taste
Pinch nutmeg
$^1/_4$ cup honey from stingless bees
1 12-oz. can Coca-Cola
Roasted bee larvae, to garnish (optional)

Wash the pork loin and dry with a paper towel. Cover with salt and pepper.

Place oil in a deep pot and heat oil to smoking point. Add pork loin and sear over high heat, turning to brown on all sides, about 8 to 12 minutes.

When evenly browned, add the spices, turning until pork loin is well coated. Add the honey, cover, and reduce heat. Let simmer until the honey liquid is absorbed.

Remove pork, retaining juices in pot, slice, and return sliced pork to pot with the Coca-Cola. Cook, covered, for approximately 30 minutes, until meat is well glazed. Serve with roasted bee larvae, if desired.

Leaf-Footed Bug Pizza

Illustration, p. 69

$^1/_2$ pound wheat flour

4 eggs

1 pinch bread yeast

1 pinch salt

2 tablespoons butter

$^1/_3$ pound leaf-footed bugs, frozen or live

2 tablespoons olive oil

$^1/_2$ pound mozzarella cheese

$^3/_4$ pound tomatoes

Salt, to taste

Pepper, to taste

herbs (thyme, marjoram, bay leaves, oregano), to taste

Preheat oven to 300°F.

Place the flour in a mixing bowl and stir in the eggs, one at a time, to form dough. Add a pinch of salt and a pinch of bread yeast and knead the dough thoroughly. Dough should rise minimally while preparing other ingredients.

Roll out pizza dough to the desired thickness. Grease a baking sheet or pizza pan with the butter and sprinkle with flour. Place the pizza dough on the greased cooking sheet.

If using frozen bugs, thaw ahead of time. If using live bugs, fry them in the oil.

Shred cheese and spread generously over the dough.

Boil some water and blanch the tomatoes for 1 minute. Take the tomatoes out and remove the skin, which should separate easily.

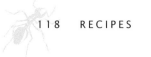

Place the skinned tomatoes in a bowl and mash with a fork, adding salt and pepper. Spread on top of the cheese.

Lay the bugs evenly over the tomato sauce. Sprinkle the pizza with the aromatic herbs and bake in the oven until cheese and crust are brown.

Sauces

Stink Bugs in Green Sauce

This sauce, like the stink bug itself, is peculiar yet exquisite. Use sparingly,
as the habaneros give it much heat!

$^1\!/_4$ pound roasted stink bugs
$^1\!/_2$ pound tomatillos
4 habanero chilies
$^1\!/_4$ medium onion, quartered
1 garlic clove
Marjoram, to taste
3–5 cilantro leaves, to taste
Bay leaves, to taste
1 avocado
Salt, to taste
Pepper, to taste

Place the tomatillos, chilies, onion, garlic, marjoram, bay leaves, cilantro, and
the avocado (*do not add* salt, which will cause the sauce to turn black) in the
blender and liquefy. Add the roasted stink bugs and liquefy. Place mixture in a
bowl and use as an accompaniment to other cooked dishes or tacos. Provide salt
and pepper to be added individually to taste after serving.

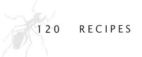

Roasted Stink Bug and Chili Sauce

6 guajillo chilies

20 tomatillos

$^1/_2$ onion

4 cloves garlic

$^1/_4$ pound roasted stink bugs

$^1/_8$ teaspoon salt

4 tablespoons peanut oil

Marjoram, to taste

Thyme, dried, to taste

Preheat oven to 450°F. Place the deveined chilies on a baking sheet and roast until soft. Place the roasted chilies and the tomatillos in a pot with enough water to cover and bring to a boil. Lower heat and simmer briefly. Remove, place in a blender with the garlic, onion, and roasted stink bugs, and liquefy.

Heat the peanut oil in a frying pan and fry the blended sauce. Add marjoram, thyme, and salt to taste. Delicious for dressing other dishes.

Leaf-Footed Bug Salsa

This traditional recipe from the town of Santiago de Anaya in the state of Hidalgo comes by way of biologist Cristina Mayorga, a native of that area. I've included it here for its exquisite and delicate pumpkinlike flavor.

$^1/_3$ **pound leaf-footed bugs**
6 ancho chilies
2 garlic cloves
Salt, to taste

Roast the garlic with the chilies. Separately roast the leaf-footed bugs (these are best when used in the nymph state).

In a mortar, mash the garlic and salt, then add the chilies, adding water to mix well. Finally, add the roasted bugs and mash all together. Place the mixture in a serving bowl. Ideal as a dip with tortilla chips.

Wasp Sauce for Meat

A-1 sauce has nothing on this divine dressing for fillet mignon, chicken breasts, or other meats.

$1/2$ stick of butter, optional
2 pounds larvae or pupae of bees and wasps, or combination
1 cup olive oil
$1/2$ cup white wine vinegar
Ground pepper, to taste
Ground mustard, to taste
Ground cloves, to taste
Ground cumin, to taste
Powdered bouillon, to taste
$1/8$ teaspoon salt

Roast the larvae and/or pupae, or heat the butter in a skillet and fry them, as desired.

Place the cooked larvae and/or pupae in a blender or food processor, along with the olive oil, vinegar, spices, bouillon, and salt. Blend until thick, and place in a small bowl to be served with the main course.

Desserts

Chicatana Empanadas

These sweet little ant turnovers make delightful snacks.

1 cup water
1 cup granulated sugar
$\frac{1}{2}$ pound ants, ground or whole
$\frac{1}{2}$ teaspoon pectin
1 cup flour to sprinkle
1 pound puff pastry dough
1 egg white, beaten, for pasting
1 egg yolk, beaten, for brushing

To prepare the filling, place the sugar and one cup of water in a pan and bring to a steady boil until it reaches a honeylike consistency. Add the ground or whole ants, and stir until a gel forms. Remove from heat and let cool. Stir in the pectin and set aside.

Preheat oven to 300°F.

Sprinkle flour on a pastry board, and roll out the pastry dough to a thickness of 1/4 inch. Use a round cookie cutter, between 2 and 3 inches in diameter, or a drinking glass with a floured rim, and cut circles out of the rolled out dough.

Place some of the filling in the center of each dough circle. Spread a bit of egg white around the top edge of each circle. Fold in half to form a half moon and press outside edge with a fork to seal. Brush with egg yolk.

Place on a greased cookie sheet about an inch apart. Bake at 300°F until golden brown.

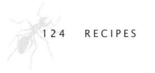

Bee Delights

$^1/_2$ pound larvae and pupae of bees or wasps
1 stick butter
$^1/_2$ cup bee or wasp honey
Cinnamon, to taste
Cardamom, to taste
Pinch of nutmeg

Heat the butter in a frying pan and fry the larvae and pupae.

Place in a serving dish. Cover with the honey and sprinkle with cinnamon, cardamom, and nutmeg, to taste. This makes for a delicious and nutritious dessert.

Kisses from the Virgin

1 pound honey from stingless bees
4 cups whey
2 tablespoons butter
cellophane to wrap candies

Slowly dissolve the honey in the whey, stirring gently until it has a dense consistency and is the color of light coffee.

Place in a saucepan over low heat and cook until it reaches a gumlike consistency.

Butter a tray or cookie sheet and spoon the honey–whey mixture onto a greased surface. Allow to cool in the refrigerator. Form by teaspoonfuls into one-inch balls. Wrap individually in cellophane.

Babinga Chocolate Cups

5 eggs

1 cup granulated sugar

1 dozen ladyfingers

$^2/_3$ pound mealworms, roasted and ground

$^1/_2$ pound baking chocolate, grated

$^3/_4$ cup dry sherry

Cherries in syrup, to garnish

Seperate the egg yolks from the egg whites. Beat the egg yolks and the sugar with a whisk until the mixture thickens enough to fall back in a ribbon when the whisk is lifted away.

In a separate bowl, beat the egg whites until they are stiff enough to form soft peaks. Fold the egg whites into the egg yolks.

Crush the ladyfingers and place in a bowl with the ground mealworms and grated chocolate and stir gently until mixed. Place in dessert cups, bake for 10 minutes at 225°F, remove from oven, and let sit for 1 hour. Add one teaspoon sherry per serving and let settle. The finished dessert will be two shades of coffee. Garnish each serving with 1 or more cherries. Delicious!

Ek Cakes

Ek is the Mayan word for star, and is also the name of the wasp Brachygastra azteca. Begin your morning with this tasty breakfast. Again, honey bee honey can be substituted for the wasp honey if necessary.

4 tablespoons butter, for creaming
2 eggs
1 cup whole wheat flour, sifted
$^1/_2$ cup wasp honey
$^1/_2$ cup sour milk
4 tablespoons butter, for cooking and dotting
2 tablespoons vanilla
1 teaspoon baking powder

Place the 4 tablespoons butter in a bowl and allow to reach room temperature.

In a separate bowl, whisk the eggs. Add the eggs to the butter and cream together thoroughly. Add the sifted flour and baking powder, the honey, and sour milk. Beat well until thickened. Stir in the vanilla.

Turn the oven on low and put plates in the oven to warm them.

Grease the bottom of a frying pan and set over low heat. When butter is melted and pan is hot place 1 ladle of the batter in the pan. When edges are cooked and bubbles appear on surface, flip pancake and cook other side. Check pancake underside by lifting with spatula, and remove when underside is golden brown. Place on a hot plate. Place a square of butter on each and top with more honey, to taste. Repeat until batter is finished. Serve each pancake fresh and hot, or keep a growing stack waiting in your prewarmed oven.

Chicatan Flan

"Chicatanas," leafcutter ants, are the ideal species for this elegant dessert, but others will do quite nicely, too.

¹/₂ pound ants, fried in butter
2 pounds granulated sugar
3 eggs
2 cups milk
1 package vanilla custard
Pinch nutmeg

Place 1 pound of the granulated sugar in a pan, over heat, stirring constantly so as not to burn, and allow to caramelize. (Use care not to burn yourself; this is a very hot process.) Cover the bottom of the mold with the caramelized sugar.

Place the eggs, milk, vanilla custard, and remaining sugar in a blender or food processor and blend. Add the butter-fried ants to the liquid ingredients.

Place the combined ingredients in the sugar-coated mold. Place the mold in a pan large enough to fill with water so that the water covers the outside of the mold but does not flow over into the mold. Bring the water to a boil, lower heat and maintain low boil for 1 hour or more, until set.

When flan is set, remove mold from water pan, and release onto a serving dish before it cools. Enjoy cooled as a dessert.

Alternative cooking method: A pressure cooker with a grill may also be used. Place water on the bottom of the pot, then the grill, and over this the filled mold. Cover tightly. Cook for 20 minutes over low heat, not letting the steam escape. Let the pot cool before uncovering. Serve cooled.

Honey of the Virgin Buñuelos

Buñuelos are a kind of thin Mexican fried dough, made unique when drizzled with the honey of stingless bees.

Honey from stingless bees, to taste
1 pound flour, or more as needed
1 egg
$^1/_2$ cup anise tea
$^1/_2$ teaspoon baking soda
1 pound butter, to fry
flour, for rolling

In a mixing bowl, combine the flour with the egg, anise tea, and baking soda, stirring constantly. Form a dough that holds together and does not stick to your hands, adding flour in small amounts as needed.

Cover and chill in the refrigerator for 1 hour.

Once chilled, divide and form into one-inch balls. Dust pastry board with flour and roll out each ball, extremely thinly, so they do not absorb too much fat when fried.

Heat butter in a frying pan. Fry dough circles one at a time, until browned. Drain on paper towels.

Serve whole or in pieces. Drizzle with honey of the virgin.

Indonesian Mealworm Bars

²/₃ pound mealworms
²/₃ pound granulated sugar
Ground cinnamon, to taste
Pinch of ground cloves
Pinch of ground cumin
4 tablespoons butter
1 sheet waxed paper

Arrange the mealworms to cover the bottom of a buttered baking sheet and set aside.

Place the sugar in a sauce pan over medium-low heat and stir until the sugar takes on a browned color. Add spices to taste. Cover the worms with the sugar while it is still hot (this will cook them).

Let cool until sugar hardens, then cut into rectangles or squares, or other interesting shapes. Place on waxed paper and delight in the flavor of these tasty and nutritious sweets.

Bee Bars

$^1/_2$ pound bee or wasp larvae and pupae

1 pound granulated sugar

4 tablespoons butter, plus additional to grease baking sheet

4 tablespoons finely chopped macadamia nuts

$^1/_2$ cup finely chopped walnuts

4 tablespoons finely chopped almonds

4 tablespoons finely chopped pine nuts

Ground cloves, to taste

Ground cinnamon, to taste

Melt the butter in a saucepan over low heat and brown the larvae and pupae. Mix together with the nuts and spices.

Place the granulated sugar in a pan over medium heat, stirring constantly, until it caramelizes.

Grease a baking sheet with butter and coat the bottom with the hot, caramelized sugar. Spread the remaining ingredients uniformly over sugar. Allow to cool and harden, cut into squares, and place on waxed paper.

Honeyed Coffee Cake

$^1/_2$ cups granulated sugar

1 cup milk

$^3/_4$ pound honey

3 eggs

1 teaspoon ground cinnamon

1 teaspoon ground ginger

$^1/_2$ teaspoon ground aniseed

1 teaspoon ground cloves

1 cup chopped walnuts

1 cup Kirsch or brandy

Grated rind of 3 oranges

$2^1/_2$ cups flour

3 level tablespoons baking powder

Preheat oven to 300°F.

Place the sugar, milk, and honey in a double boiler and heat until well blended and warm. Let cool.

In a small bowl beat the eggs. Whisk in the spices and add the nuts, Kirsch or brandy, and grated orange rind. Mix in the cooled liquid.

In a separate bowl, mix the sifted flour with the baking powder. Add this to the egg mixture a little at a time, beating gently. Continue until well combined.

Pour into greased cake pan and bake for approximately 40 minutes until a knife stuck into the center comes out clean.

Turron

Turron is a Spanish dessert that is something like a cross between fruitcake and meringue, hard and crunchy with plenty of dried fruits.

1¹/₂ cups honey
2¹/₂ tablespoons water
¹/₂ pound granulated sugar
2 egg whites
1 pound toasted almonds
¹/₂ pound toasted hazelnuts
Grated rind of 5 lemons
assorted dried fruits, chopped (figs, dates,
     pineapples, cherries, prunes, etc.)

Heat the honey in a double boiler, stirring constantly with a wooden spoon, until it is a golden color, about 1 hour.

Bring the water to a boil and add the sugar, stirring over medium heat until mixture thickens.

In a mixing bowl, beat the egg whites until soft peaks form when the whisk is pulled away. Add the heated honey and the nuts, stirring constantly, until mixture reaches a spongy consistency. Add this to the sugar–water mixture and continue stirring over medium heat, testing periodically, until a small amount placed in water forms a hard mass.

Add the dried fruits and the grated lemon peel and stir.

Place in molds and cover with Nevada crackers. Cool in refrigerator, turn out of molds, and serve.

Places to Purchase Edible Insects

(most of these companies carry crickets and mealworms)

Armstrong's Cricket Farm
P.O. Box 125
West Monroe, LA 71294-0125
For orders: 1-800-345-8778
For inquiries: (318) 387-6000

Bassetts Cricket Ranch
353 North Lover's Lane
Visalia, CA 93292
For inquiries: 1-800-634-2445

Beneficial Insect Company
555 Skyway
Paradise, California 95969
For inquiries: 916-472-3715

Fluker's Cricket Farm
Box 378
Baton Rouge, LA 70821
For inquiries: 1-800-735-8537

Grubco, Inc.
P.O. Box 15001
Hamilton, OH 45015
For orders: 1-800-222-3563
For inquiries: (513) 874-5881

Hotlix Co. (insect snacks)
179 Palmeroy
Pismo Beach, CA 93449
Phone: (805) 773-1942 or 1-800-
EAT-WORM

Hurst Cricket Farm
Attn: Mike Young
P.O. Box 212
Savannah, TN 38372
For inquiries: (901) 925-4019

Rainbow Mealworms
123 E. Spruce Street
Compton, CA 90224
For inquiries: 1-800-777-9676
or (310) 635-1494

Waxworms, Inc.
P.O. Box 333
Cameron, WI 54822
For inquires: (715) 924-2777

Entomophagy Books and Other Publications of Interest

Butterflies in my Stomach
by Ronald Taylor
Woodbridge Press Publishing Co.
P.O. Box 209
Santa Barbara, CA 93101

Dreadful Delicacies
by Mary Ann Clayton
Longstreet Press, Inc.
2140 Newmarket Parkway
Suite 118
Marietta, GA 30067

Entertaining with Insects
by Ronald Taylor and Barbara Carter
Salutek Publishing Co.
5375 Crescent Drive
Yorba Linda, CA 92687

The Food Insects Newsletter
Dr. Florence V. Dunkel, Editor
Department of Entomology
324 Leon Johnson Hall
University of Montana
Bozeman, MT 59717-0302
Phone: 406-994-5065
Fax: 406 994-6029
E-mail: ueyd@msu.oscs.montana.edu

Instinctive Nutrition
by Severen Schaeffer.
Celestial Arts
Box 7327
Berkeley, CA 94707

Insects as a Source of Protein in the
  Future (in Spanish)
by Dr. Juliet Ramos-Elorduy
Limusa Ed.
Instituto de Biología UNAM,
  Mexico
Apdo. Postal 70-153
04510 Mexico D.F.
Fax: (5) 550-0164
e-mail:
  relorduy@mail.ibiologia.unam.mx

Edible Insects in Ancient Mexico: An
  Ethnoentomological Study (in
  Spanish)
by Dr. Julieta Ramos-Elorduy and
  José Manuel Pino Moreno
ED AGT
Instituto de Biología UNAM,
  Mexico
Apdo. Postal 70-153
04510 Mexico D.F.
Fax: (5) 550-0164
e-mail:
  relorduy@mail.ibiologia.unam.mx

Special Events and Places of Interest

The Bug Bowl
Purdue University
Entomology Department
West Lafayette, IN 47907-1185
Phone: 765-494-4568
Contact: Tom Turpin, Coordinator
Special events: Food insects, cock-
    roach races, cricket spitting,
    insects as art and more (spring)

Buggette Fest
Eagle Bluff Environmental Learning
    Center
Route 2 Box 156
Lanesboro, MN 93449
Phone: 507-467-2437
Fax: 507-467-3583
Contact: Lolly Melander
Special events: Insect eating

Buffalo Museum of Science
Division of Invertebrate Zoology
1020 Humboldt parkway
Buffalo, NY 14211-1293
Phone 716-896-5200
Contact: Wayne K. Gall

Insect Horror Film Festival
Entomology Department
411 Science 2
Iowa State University
Aimes, IA 50010
Phone: 515-294-7400
Contact: Entomology Club president

Montreal Insectarium and Botanical
   Gardens
4581 rue Sherbrooke Est
Montreal, Quebec H1X 2B2
Canada
Phone: 514-872-0663 or 514-872-
   1453
Contact: Marjolaine Grioux
Special events: Annual insect eating
   festival (February)

San Francisco Zoo
Insect Zoo
1 Zoo Road
San Francisco, CA 94132
Phone: 415-753-7080
Contact: Leslie Saul-Gershenz

Bibliography

Andary C., Motte-Florac E., Ramos-Elorduy J., and Privat A. (1997) "Chemical screening: Updated methodology applied to medicinal insects." *Healing, Yesterday and Today, Tomorrow?* Vol. 3, Ethnomedicine Library, Erga Edizioni, Italy.

Bahuchet S. (1978) *Introduction à la ethnoécologie des pygemées Aka de la Lobaye Empire Centre African.* Ph.D. thesis, Ecole Supérieure d'Hautes Etudes.

Beckerman S. (1979) "La abundancia de proteinas en la Amazonia: Una respuesta a Gross." *Amazonia Pervana* 3(6): 91–126.

Blake A. E. and Wagner M. R. (1987) "Collection and consumption of Pandora moth *(Coloradia pandora lindsleyi)* (Lepidoptera-Saturniidae) larvae by Owens Valles and Mono Lake Paiutes." *Bull. Ent. Soc. Amer.* 33(1):139–141.

Bodenheimer N. (1951) *Insects as Human Food* (Junk: The Hague), 239.

Bourges R. H. (1984) *Panorma de la Nutrición y de la alimentación en México.*

(Mexico City: National Autonomous University in Mexico), 27–48.

DeFoliart G. R. (1975) Insects as sources of protein. *Bull. Ent. Soc. Amer.* 21(3): 161–163.

———. (1989) "The human use of insects as food and as animal feed." *Bull. Ent. Soc. Amer.* 35:22–35.

DeFoliart G. R., Finke M.D., and Sunde M. L. (1982) "Potential value of the mormom cricret (Orthoptera-Tettigonidae) harvested as a high protein feed for poultry." *J. Econ. Ent.* 75:848–852.

Dufour D. L. (1987) "Insects as food: A case study from the northwest Amazon." *Am. Anthropol.* 89:383–397.

Evans M. I. (1993) "Conservation by commercialization." *Food and Nutrition in the Tropical Forest: Biocultural Interactions and Applications to Development.* UNESCO, 815-828.

FAO (1964) "Protein at the heart of the world food problem." *World Food Problems,* Vol. 5.

FAO/OMS/UNU (1985) *Necesidades de Eearergia y de Proteinus.* (Serie de informes térenicos 724). OMS, p. 220.

FAO/WHO (1965) *Protein Requirements.* FAO Nutr. Mtg. Rep. Ser. 37.

Fernández V. G. (1987) *Evaluation of an edible resource native to Lagos Alcalinos Insecta-Hemiptera-Corixidae y Notonectidae.* Ph.D. thesis, National Autonomous University in Mexico.

Fisher et al. (1979) *Recent Advances in Animal Nutrition* (London: Butterworths), 167.

Gelfand M. (1971) *Diet and Tradition in an African Culture* (Edinburg: G. F. Brock), 248.

Gibbons A. (1991) "Small is beautiful: Microlivestock for the Third World." *Science* 253–378.

Gómez P. A., Hato T. R., and Collin A. (1961) "Production of animal proteins in the Congo." *Bull. Agri. Congo* 52(4):689–815.

Hernández O. M. C. (1987) *Elaboración de un dulce a partir del gusano amarillo de la harina*. Ph.D thesis, Q. F. B. O., 74.

Horwitz W. (1975) *Official Methods of Analysis of the Association of Official Analytical Chemists*. Association of Official Analytical Chemists (Washington, U.S.A.), 1094.

Hunn E. S. (1977) *The Classification of Discontinuities in Nature Tzeltal Folk Zoology* (New York: Acamdemic Press), 363.

Ichponani J. and Malek N. (1971) "Evaluation of de-oiled silk worm pupae meal as protein sources in chicken rations." *Br. Poul. Sci.* 12:231–234.

Jones J. G. W. (1973) *The Biological Efficiency of Protein Production* (Cambridge: University Press), 107.

Jones K. T. and Madsen D. B. (1991) "Further experiments in native food procurement." *Utah Archaeol* 68–77.

Kitsa K. (1989) "Contribution of edible insects to the improvement of diet in the Western Kasai of Zaire." *Zaire-Afrique* 239:511–519.

Kodonki K., Leclerq G., and Gaudin-Harding F. (1987) "Vitamin estimations of three edible species of Attacidae caterpillars from Zaire." *Int. J. Vit. Nutr. Res.* 57:333–334.

Kodonki K., Leclerq M., Bourgeay-Caussem M., Pascaud A., and Gaudin-Harding F. (1987) "Nutritional value of Attacidae caterpillars from Zaire." *Nutritive. Cah. Nutr. Diet.* 22(6):47883–47885.

Kok R. (1983) "The production of insects for human food (*Stegobium paniceum*)." *J. Can. Inst. Food Sci. Technol.* 16:5-18.

Ladron de Guevara O., Padilla P., Garcia G. M., Pino J. M., and Ramos-Elorduy J. (1996) "Amino acid determination in some edible Mexican insects." *Aminoacids* 9:161–173.

Lawtie R. A. (1970) *Protein as Human Food* (London: Butterworths), 396.

Leleup P. and Daems A. (1969) "Nutritious caterpillars of Kwago." *J. Atric. Trop. Bot. Appl.* 16(1):1–21.

Loomis R. (1986) "Agriculatural systems." *Investigación y Ciencia Ed. Sci. Am.* 2:76–84.

Malaisse F. and Parent G. (1980) "Edible Caterpillars of Zaire." *Nat. Belges.* 61(1):2–24.

McDonald P., Edwards R. A., and Greenhalg J. E. (1982) *Animal Nutrition* (n.p.: Longman; n.p.: John Wiley & Sons), 543.

Meyer-Rochow V. B. (1973) "Edible insects in three different ethnic groups of Papua and New Guinea." *Amer. J. Clinical. Nutr.* 26:663–677.

Mitsuhoshi J. (1980) *Edible Insects of the World* (in Japanese) (Tokyo: Kokinshoin Kanda), 270.

Muyay T. (1981) *Les Insectes Comme Aliments de l"Homme.* CEEBA publication, series 2, 69:177.

Nkuoka E. (1987) "Edible insects in Central African societies." *Muntu Rev. Sci. and Cult. du CICIBA* 6:171–178.

Pereira N. (1974) *Panorama da Alimentaçao Indigena: Comidas Bebidas y Toxicos na Amazonia Brasilcira* (Rio de Janeiro: Livraria Sao Jose), 442.

Pimentel D. (1980) "Energy and land constraints in food protein production." *Science* 190:754–761.

Pimentel D. et al (1977) "Pesticides, insects in foods, and cosmetic standards." *Bioscience* 27(3):178–185.

Posey D. (1980) "Sobre los grupos amerindios." *América Indigena* 40(1):105–120.

Quin P. (1959) *Foods and Feeding Habits of the Pedi.* Ph.D. thesis, Witwaterstand University.

Ramos-Elorduy J. (1982) *Insects as a Source of Protein in the Future* (Mexico City: Editorial Limusa), 144.

————. (1984) *Los insectos como un recurso actual y potencial*. Institute of Geography, National Autonomous University in Mexico, 120–139.

————. (1987) "Are insects edible? Man's attitude toward the eating of insects." In *Food Deficiency Studies and Perspectives*. UNESCO, 78–83.

————. (1990) "Edible insects barbarism or solution to the hunger problem in Possey D. A." *Ethnobiology Implications and Applications*. Proc. of the First Int. Congress of Ethnobiology Belem, Brazil 7:151–158.

————. (1993). "Insects in the diets of the tropical forest people in Mexico." In *Food and Nutrition in the Tropical Forest Biocultural Interactions and Applications to Development*. UNESCO, 205–212.

————. (1996) "Rôle des insects dans l'alimentation en Forêt Tropicale." *L'Alimentation en Foret Tropicale*. UNESCO, 1:371–381.

————. (1998) "Importance of edible insects in the nutrition and economy of the people living in the rural area." *J. Ecol. Food Nutr.* (in press).

————. (1998) "Insects as a means of national identity." *Ehtnobiol. Hum. Wel.* (in press).

————. (1998) "Insects as intermediate biotransformers." *Hum. Ecol.* (in press).

————. (1998) "Importance of edible insects in the nutrition and economy of people living in the rural areas of Mexico." *J. Ecol. Food Nutr.* (in press).

————. (1998) "Insects as intermediary biotransformers for obtaining proteins." *Hum. Ecol.* (in press).

————. (1998) "Insects: A new feasible sustainable alternative?" *J. Ecol. Food Nutr.* (in press).

Ramos-Elorduy J. and Bourges H. (1977) "Nutritional value of some edible insects of the world." *Ann. Inst. de Biol. UNAM Ser. Zool.* 48(1):167–186.

Ramos-Elorduy J., Bourges H., and Pino J. M. (1982) "Nutritional value and protein quality of some edible insects of Mexico." *Fol. Ent. Mex.* 53:111–118.

Ramos-Elorduy J., Bourges H., Martinez N., and Pino J. M. (1986) "Bio test REP and UNP on a rat Wistar to estimate the protein quality of three edible insects of Mexico." *Rev. Tec. Alim.* 20(4):24.

Ramos-Elorduy J. and Conconi M. (1993) "Resemblance of the techniques for exploit some edible insect species in different ethnic groups all over the world." *II Int. Cong. Ethnobiol. Abstracts* 141.

Ramos-Elorduy J., Levieux J., and Lenoir A. (1992) "Possibilitiés de renforcement des fondations chez deux especés de fourmis de'intéret économique. Premiers resultats (Liometopum. Hymenoptera. Formicidae)." *Anls. Soc. Ent. Fr. (NS)* 28(2): 215–219.

Ramos-Elorduy J., Morales J., Pino J. M., and Nieto Z. (1988) "Contents of thiamine, riboflavin, and niacin of some edible insects of Mexico." *Rev. Tec. Alim.* 22: 76–81.

Ramos-Elorduy J. and Pino, J. M. (1993). "Biogeographical aspects of some edible insects from Mexico." *II Int. Cong. Ethnobiol. Abstracts* 43.

Ramos-Elorduy J., Pino J. M., Escamilla E. P., Lagunez J. O., and Ladréon de Guevara O. (1997) "Nutritional value of edible insects from the state of Oaxaca, Mexico." *Journ. Foods Comp. Analys.* 10(2):149–157.

Ramos-Elorduy J. M., Pino M., and Gonzalez O. (1980) *"In vitro* digestibility of some edible insects of Mexico." *Fol. Ent. Mex.* 49:118.

Ramos-Elorduy J., Pino J. M., and Romero S. (1988) "Determination of the nutritive value of some species of edible insects of the state of Puebla." *Ann. Inst. de Biol. UNAM Ser. Zool.* 58(1):355–372.

Ramos-Elorduy J. et al. (1984) "Protein content of some edible insects in Mexico." *J. Ethnobiol.* 4:61–72.

Redford K. H. and Dorea J. G. (1984) "The nutritional value of invertebrates with emphasis on ants and termites as food for mammals." *J. Zool.* 203:385–395.

Ruddle K. (1973) "The Human use of insects examples from the Yukpa." *Biotrópica* 5(2):94–101.

Schurr K. (1972) "Insects as a major protein source in sewage lagoon biomass useable as animal food." *Proc. Entomol. Soc. Amer. N.C.B.* 27:135–137.

Smith H. S., (1992) *Global Biodiversity: Status of the Earth's Living Resources* (London: Chapman and Hall), 594.

Sutton M. (1988) *Insects as Food Aboriginal Entomophagy in the Great Basin* (n.p.: Ballena Press), 115.

Taylor R. (1975) *Buttlerflies in my Stomach* (Santa Barbara: Woodbridge Press).

Toledo V. (1998) "Entobiologia para un desarrolol sustentable: Hacia una nueva etapa de la investigación en México." In *Etnobiologia en el Conocimiento y Conservacion de los Recursos Natruales y Culturales* (in press).

Van der Waal B. C. W. (1994) "The importance of grasshoppers as traditional food in villages in northern Trans vaal South Africa." *Fourth Int. Cong. Ethnobiol. Abstracts.* Lucknow, India, 140.

Vand der Meer J. C. (1965) "Insects eaten by the Karo-Batak people." *Entomologische Berichten* 25(6):101–107.

Weaver N. and Weaver E. C. (1981) "Beekeeping with the stingless bee *Melipona beeckei* by the Yucatan Maya." *Bee World* 62:7-19.

Wilson E. O. (1985) "The biological diversity crisis: A challenge to science." *Issues Sci. Technol* 2:20-29.

———. (1987) "The little things that run the world: the importance and con-servation of invertebrates." *Conserv. Biol.* 1:344–346.

Index of Scientific Names

Following is a list of the insects that figure prominently in the recipes and elsewhere in this book. Where more than one species is listed, these are alternatives that are known to be edible. You may substitute local insects for those that appear in these recipes, but only do so after verifying with an expert that the species in question is edible.

Agave Billbug: *Scyphophorus acupunctatus*

Ant: *Liometopum occidentale, L. apiculatum, Pogonomyrmex barbatus, Formica excestoides, F. obscuripes*

Backswimmer: *Notonecta unifasciata, N. undulata*

Bee: *Apis mellifera, Bombus occidentalis*

Black witch moth: *Ascalapha odorata. Saturniidae* sp. can be substituted

Boll weevil: *Anthonomus grandis*

Corn earworm: *Heliothis zea*

Cricket: *Acheta domestica*

Damselfly: *Enallagma praevarum, Ischnura verticalis, I. denticollis*

Diving Beetle: *Dytiscus mexicanus*

Dobsonfly: *Corydalus cornutus*

Dragonfly: *Anax junius, Aeshna multicolor, Perithemis tenera*

Giant water bug: *Lethocerus americanus*

Grasshopper: *Melanoplus femur-rubrum, M. differentialis, M. atlantis, M. mexicanus, Sphenarium histrio, S. purpurascens, Schistocerca americana, S. vaga vaga, S. shoshone*

Leaf-footed bug: *Thasus gigas, Sephina grayi, S. vinula, Piezogaster calculator, P. idecorus*

Leafcutting ant: *Atta texana, A. mexicana, A. cephalotes*

Mealworm: *Tenebrio molitor*

Nopal worm: *Laniifera cyclades*

Paper wasp: *Polistes instabilis, P. major, P. Aphanilopterus canadensis*

Red agave worm: *Xyleutes redtenbachi*

Stingless bee: *Melipona beecheii, M. interrupta*

Stink bug: *Euschistus sp., Brochymena arborea, B. tenebrosa, Edessa sp.*

Stonefly: *Pteronarcys sp.*

Tree worm: Cerambycidae sp., Buprestidae sp., Passalidae sp.

Treehopper: *Hoplophorion monograma, Ceresa bubalus*

Wasp: *Vespula pennsylvanica, V. germanica, Brachygastra azteca, B. mellifica*

Water boatman: *Corisella edulis, C. mercenaria, Krizousacorixa femorata, K. azteca, Callicorixa vulnerata, Hesperocorixa interrupta, Graptocorixa californica*

White agave worm: *Aegiale (acentrocneme) hesperiasis*